Praise for *Hypnosis & Counselling*
Cancer and other Chron

CW00519962

I feel that I have on my desk here possibly one
written to date on the true therapeutic properties
of serious and life threatening illness. I found it one of those books that I
could not put down until completed. It is written in a very clear, uncluttered
style with the minimum of unnecessary jargon and unpronounceable words.
It is interesting and full of fascinating information into the bargain.

For those of us who may find it somewhat difficult to convince doctors of
our valid place amongst the Health professionals, this book gives clear,
supported, well researched material to endorse our claim. Through its clarity
of text and also its many intensely interesting case studies, this book, from
cover to cover, portrays the true value of hypnosis in the treatment
of chronic illness, even life threatening illness. It is a book not only for us
as hypnotherapists but also would be of great value to all who work in the
health field related to the care of people with chronic and life threatening
illness. I find this a compelling book in every way and am pleased to
recommend it to you.

David Slater, The Hypnotherapist

With this book, David Frank and Bernard Mooney have made a valuable
contribution to the corpus of Complementary and Alternative Medicine
(CAM). Given that standard medical practices within the National Health
Service cannot meet the needs of the populace, one can safely conclude
that the whole of the United Kingdom would benefit should a copy of this
book be placed in every doctor's surgery where both medical practitioners
and patients could be exposed to the principles of this therapeutic approach
to effecting cures for all kinds of ailments including cancer.

June Adams

This is a very informative, interesting and very readable publication and
should be on the bookshelves of anyone involved in treating those with
chronic illness, those people who have a chronic illness or in fact anybody
who is interested in protecting themselves from contracting such illness.

Mark Storey, Clinical Hypnotherapist, Positive Solution Training
& Development

There are very few books on the subject of hypnosis and hypnotherapy that are of equal value and interest to both practitioners and the general public alike. This book is undoubtedly one of them.

A succinct work of substance, this book delivers its agreeably positive message in a most accessible fashion. Although the authors' primary interest is clearly in highlighting the value of hypnosis as an essential (yet woefully neglected) component in the overall treatment of cancer and chronic illness, their findings may clearly be extended to the entire gamut of human suffering.

Offering an overview of the major (psycho) therapeutic approaches, the authors present a compelling argument that hypnotic elements are present in all of them. In the process, they also go some considerable way towards elevating the status of hypnotherapy to its rightful position on a par with all other methodologies
.

Liberally salted with actual case histories that serve to whet the appetite for further study, this book will both stimulate and inspire readers on either side of the therapeutic relationship. I unreservedly recommend it to all who are interested in the improvement of their own lives or the wellbeing of others.

William Broom, Chief Executive & Registrar,
The General Hypnotherapy Standards Council

The authors of this volume, David Frank and Bernard Mooney. Ph.D., work from the theoretical premise that many illnesses, including cancer, that have been traditionally viewed as organic or purely physical are, in fact, stress-related problems that can be effectively treated with counseling, and hypnosis in particular. The authors suggest that hypnosis and counseling extend beyond the often identified application of treating symptoms, in some cases, to providing the primary tool to effect a cure or complete remission in chronic illness. I find this assertion both bold and refreshing because it builds on the premise that human beings have the mental capacity to impact positively their health and well being. This position does not negate or even suggest that people should avoid more traditional, mainstream Western medical treatments, but rather that we should approach with open minds the question of identifying true curative factors in recovery from chronic illness.

A major strength of this book is that, whenever possible, the authors attempt to describe the specifics of the hypnotic interventions used in the case material. This is a major bonus for practicing clinicians. Although the use of hypnotic approaches is considered atheoretical, I found it useful to highlight the congruence between person-centered psychotherapy and clinical hypnosis. This book is very readable and jargon free. I would suggest it as most suited for beginning students of hypnosis, lay persons interested in learning how hypnosis and self-hypnosis could be of benefit in dealing with chronic illness, and a good introduction for other healthcare providers who may not be aware of the potential uses of hypnosis in the medical field.

American Journal of Clinical Hypnosis

This is the book I wish I'd had the ability to write. Not only do the authors set out a very clear case for the uses of counselling and particularly hypnotherapeutic techniques in healing chronic illness, they back their theories up with clinical case histories, some of which go back to the nineteenth century. While this will come as no surprise to most therapists, there are probably many sufferers of chronic illnesses who might be persuaded, by reading this book, that there is something they can do to help themselves.

The most difficult thing, particularly in the case of many cancer sufferers, is for them to believe that the mind is capable of healing the body and I believe this book may be the key to changing their beliefs. Of course, the book would have to be brought to their attention first and, to this end, perhaps self-help groups might be instrumental in guiding their participants towards it. GPs and Hospital personnel could also do their bit by recommending that their patients read this book, not only to help effect healing when a disease is contracted but also to prevent these illnesses occurring in the first place.

I particularly liked the section at the end of the book, which deals with parenting, as I, like the authors, believe that better parenting could result in fewer illnesses in later life. Altogether, a very readable, interesting and informative book which will be useful and beneficial to therapists and the general public alike.

Pat Doohan

From the beginning, the authors of this volume recognize what seasoned hypnotherapists know -everyone can be hypnotized if they want or need to be- this is especially true for people who are suffering. The authors align Erickson and Rogers as a therapeutic model by briefly discussing how each believed that the client has all the resources required for healing already within them. This is offered as a powerful attitude with which to engage in counseling and hypnosis.

Thin books, only 124 pages of text, demand more from authors. Frank and Mooney have sifted through shelves of history, research and case studies to offer a quietly compelling treatise advocating the use of hypnosis as an integral part of a comprehensive treatment plan for chronic and potentially terminal illnesses.

As part of their observations, the authors note cases that have resulted in individuals experiencing remission or cure (individuals who had been previously diagnosed as "imminently terminal") have not been given the attention deserved to such phenomena. I am planning to pass this book along to a reluctant oncologist.

Deborah Beckman M.S., LPC, NCC,
The Milton H. Erickson Foundation Newsletter

This book is significant to all those who have an interest in the ways we treat disease, arguing compellingly for the use of hypnosis with cancer patients as well as other areas of disease such as asthma, ME or chronic fatigue syndrome (myalgic encephalomyelitis) and general pain relief It also looks at the benefits of using hypnosis for such things as childbirth, stammering and many emotional health issues. This work provides crucial insight into the body's healing abilities, an insight that we cannot afford to ignore. It gives the practitioner the well-researched statistics derived from medical trials in regards to hypnosis versus such things as drug therapy, the placebo effect, psychotherapy and basic counselling.

This volume would be of particular interest to doctors, nurses, counsellors and anyone involved in the care of people with chronic or life-threatening illnesses. This could be a good introduction to the uses of hypnotherapy for practitioners who are interested in alternative and holistic therapies.

Lyndall Briggs, Vice President, Australian Society
of Clinical Hypnotherapists

I'm adding weight to the review by Lyndall Briggs published in the *Australian Journal of Clinical Hypnotherapy & Hypnosis*, having found it an absorbing book that covers so many aspects of the mind/body connection. Example after example of the uses of therapeutic Hypnosis abound. The authors have combined their skills to present evidence of how Hypnosis and Counselling can be used to affect the status of physical and emotional health. This book is a well researched offering, and is rich with references that will spur the reader to explore even further in this area.

Lyn Macintosh, ASCH

If only all doctors read this book as part of their training! Some oncologists still maintain the belief that the mind has no part in the onset of cancer and other chronic illnesses! David Frank and Bernard Mooney state that it is their intention to show how hypnotherapy can be used to discover the psychosomatic reasons for the occurrence of cancer in some people. They do this from their own case studies, and other documented evidence. They then searched for studies on the effectiveness of hypnotherapy in the treatment of cancer. (These are numerous.) They maintain that a normal healthy immune system destroys cancerous cells on a daily basis, but when an immune system is overwhelmed by fear, depression, negativity, self-hatred or suppressed anger, (the most damaging forms of stress), the will to live can be removed. Freud first described the 'unconscious death wish,' which was derided by his followers, but David Frank and Bernard Mooney explain clearly how this is a feasible hypothesis.

Some patients find death a preferable alternative to lives that are too burdensome. In some cases, when these feelings are released, the patient improves and is healed. There are a number of ways that hypnosis and counselling can help sufferers. This book is clear and easy to read by anyone who is concerned with long-term illness, and has numerous references. There is a synopsis of the history and development of hypnosis, and explanations about it, so this book is a useful introduction for counsellors and allied professionals who may be considering the use of hypnosis in their work. At the same time, it is a valuable contribution to the literature on hypnotherapy.

Hypnotherapy Now – December 2003

Psychoneuroimmunology is in essence the study of behavioural, psychological, neuroendocrinal processes and how they interrelate and impact on immunology (Reber & Reber, 2001), and this book covers just this subject in a succinct and readable manner.

This is by no means a "self-help" book that offers DIY instructions on how to solve the world's problems, but is a book by practitioners for practitioners. It is not a highly theoretical ivory tower book, but one that offers a blend of theory and a large dose of practical "how to get the job done", and it is here that one can see it is a book written by two people who get their hands dirty doing what they preach. All in all, an enjoyable, easy reading, yet highly informative book that motivates one not to lose sight of those often indirect effects of counselling and hypnosis, and how these can often have such phenomenal impact on chronic illness.

Phillip De Ronchi, B.A. Dip. Hypnotherapy. Murdoch University,
Western Australia

This volume is a serious and thoughtful discussion of the healing benefits of hypnosis in the treatment of life-threatening and chronic diseases. Written by two leading figures in the British Association for the Person Centered Approach, it carefully and considerately examines therapeutic hypnosis for matters such as childbirth, pain relief, stammering, asthma, chronic fatigue syndrome, emotional health, and more. *Hypnosis & Counselling in the Treatment of Cancer and Other Chronic Illness* is an intelligent and articulate study of this branch of alternative medicine that is suitable for professionals in the field as well as interested non-specialist general readers.

The Midwest Book Review

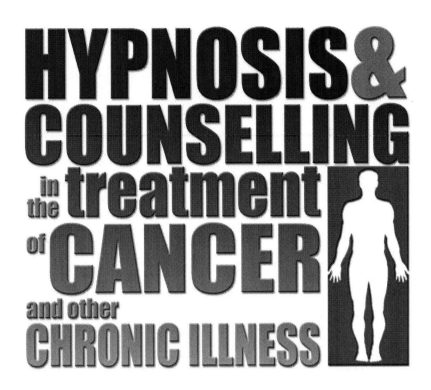

HYPNOSIS & COUNSELLING in the treatment of CANCER and other CHRONIC ILLNESS

David Frank & Bernard Mooney PhD

Crown House Publishing Limited
www.crownhouse.co.uk
www.chpus.com

First published by
Crown House Publishing Ltd
Crown Buildings
Bancyfelin, Carmarthen, Wales, SA33 5ND, UK
www.crownhouse.co.uk
and

Crown House Publishing Company, LLC
6 Trowbridge Drive, Suite 5, Bethel, CT 06801-2858, USA
www.crownhousepublishing.com

Originally published as *Hypnosis and Counselling in the
Treatment of Chronic Illness* in hardback (Original ISBN: 1899836748)

British Library Catalouging-in-Publications Data
A catalog entry for this book is available
from the British Library.

ISBN: 978-1845900809

LCCN: 2007932737

Printed in the United States of America

We would like to dedicate this book to

Doctor John Elliotson

Dr John Elliotson was from the nineteenth century. He was an imaginative, intelligent and courageous healer who published, boldly, cases from his work that were at the centre of controversy. His courage led him into trouble from the conservative medical establishment, who struck him off for a while. He was sacked from University College Hospital, London, UK, because he gave public demonstrations of mesmerism (hypnotism). Despite these set-backs, he lost no faith in himself and was finally reinstated and given full recognition by being asked to deliver the Harveian Oration.

Acknowledgments

We would like to thank the following people for their help with this book:

Mary Frank – for her encouragement and constancy in allowing us the maximum time we could have for the work

Sara Callen – for her gathering of data for us and for helpful criticism of our writing

Christian Gilson – for checking the text

Robert Gillat – for proofreading and valuable literary criticism

Bernadette McCarthy – for typing part of our manuscript

Michael Gallagher – for typing part of the manuscript

Daphne Mooney – for relevant newspaper articles and her patience during time spent on our work

Mervyn Jones – whose inspiration to us both has led to its creation

Our volunteers – who gave their permission to use their notes as our own case studies

Matthew Pearce, Bridget Shine, Helen Kinsey, Sam Hemmant and our copy editor AA for their great help with patience, courtesy and professional tenacity. Any errors they were not able to find for us are ours alone.

Table of Contents

Introduction

Hypnosis Can Treat Cancer

If hypnotherapy is so good why are the doctors not using it?

In 1953 a British Medical Association Subcommittee reported that hypnotism "is a proper subject for enquiry by the tried methods of medical research and that it should be taught far more widely than it is".[1] There are pockets of medical practice and individual practitioners who use, and have used for many years, hypnosis for a variety of successful treatments. David Waxman's book, *Hartland's Medical and Dental Hypnosis*,[2] illustrates this thoroughly. However, generally speaking, hypnosis and hypnotherapy are left to the lay practitioner.

The *New York Times* of 24 April 1988 asserted that survival rates for cancer sufferers had not markedly improved for 40 years. It was a bit of a shock to read. In certain categories there have been small improvements, but alas in some the opposite is true. This is despite all improvements in surgical techniques, the increase in chemotherapy and the improvement in the precision of radiation treatment. These improvements have decreased side effects and discomfort in general, and have led to better pain control. However, the survival rates have hardly altered.[3]

More recent statistics published in 1999 by Professor M Coleman cover 1971–1990 for England and Wales. This book, recommended by a librarian at Cancer Research, recognises 48 cancer sites. It seems that such complicated and extensive statistics need nine years to assemble and publish. We include some approximate figures to illustrate the complexity:

Cancer site	Cancer sufferers	Increase in 5-year survival rates 1971–1990
Lung	≈ 1 in 4	≈ 1%
Breast	≈ 1 in 6	≈ 13%
Colon	≈ 1 in 10	≈ 17%
Stomach	≈ 1 in 13	≈ 5%
Rectum	≈ 1 in 14	≈ 12%
Prostate	≈ 1 in 14	≈ 11%
Bladder	≈ 1 in 14	≈ 18%
Pancreas	≈ 1 in 28	≈ 1%
Skin melanoma	≈ 1 in 200	≈ 2%
Liver	≈ 1 in 200	≈ 1%
Salivary glands	≈ 1 in 400	≈ –0.1%

To claim any of these as a marked improvement seems ambitious for a period of nearly 20 years. If you have cancer of the lungs, pancreas, liver or salivary glands, improvement in survival rate is 1% or less.

Our theory is that many organic (purely physical) illnesses, including cancer, are in fact stress-related and can be effectively treated by counselling; and, as one of the therapeutic methods, *hypnotherapy* seems to be the most effective.

Susan Seliger in her book *Stop Killing Yourself*,[4] recounts the tale of a ten-year-old boy with an inoperable brain tumour. Radiation treatment did not halt the growth of the tumour. He was thought to be dying. At the Menninger Clinic, PO Box 829, Topeka, Kansas, USA, he was *taught to use his imagination* and see himself as an air force ace who attacks the planetoid (tumour) with torpedoes, each night. Eight months later, two months beyond his expected life span, improvements in his motor control were observed. Then one night, as he searched for his target, he could not find it. He told his father, "There are only some funny white spots where the planetoid is supposed to be." A CAT (computerised axial tomography) scan revealed a cluster of bony white chips, little calcium deposits. He was still alive in 1984 when Susan Seliger wrote her book. Seliger points out that today more and more of us are aware of the effect of our moods, personalities and attitudes on diseases. The name given to this profound effect is *psychoneuroimmunology*: the study of the interplay of the mind, the nervous system and the immune system. Psychotherapy can boost the human immune system and can include meditation, guided fantasy, counselling and hypnosis. We see hypnotherapy, with the use of self-hypnosis, as able to maximise the healing powers of the mind, nervous system and immune system, in combination. This book has arisen from the seed of an idea. One of us, DF, through a personal observation, saw hypnotherapy increase the life expectancy of a woman who had twice had breast cancer. This experience led to a search in the learned literature, and other sources, for evidence of the effectiveness of hypnotherapy. We found successful treatments of what most people think of as organic conditions. This suggests that cancer is often emotional and stress-related (psychosomatic). There are many examples. This book presents the most dramatic case studies taken from the quoted sources, so as to initiate a debate, and hopefully promote a change of attitudes in the medical profession on this controversial subject. People can ask their own doctor for such treatment, which is available from qualified hypnotherapists.

It is our intention to show how hypnotherapy can be used to discover the psychosomatic reasons for the occurrence of cancer in some people. We shall detail some of our own cases, where hypnosis has provided an answer to the cause of cancer. We present case studies from a variety of sources where hypnosis has been used effectively to help in the treatment of cancer.

Chapter 1

What is Hypnosis?

We hope to show in this chapter that hypnosis and what are known as hypnoidal states are a part of our everyday experience. Of course, we do not always know that we are experiencing such states when they occur. While some schools say only a small majority of people are likely to succumb to hypnosis, we believe that everyone can be hypnotised, *if they wish or need to be*.

Along the way, in our brief history of hypnotism, we introduce some of the foremost researchers and practitioners in the use of hypnosis and hypnotherapy, whose experiences will help us to gain more insight into this very real, effective and empowering phenomenon, which we believe can – used with care and the right attitude on the part of the patient – be invaluable in the promotion of growth and healing.

A Brief History of Hypnotism

Healing by trance state (hypnosis) is one of the oldest arts. Early man believed the seemingly miraculous cures, which often resulted, were the works of gods. There are few cultures, anywhere in the world, without a tradition of shamanism, voodoo or witch-doctors; and it is still a matter of common belief that some people have the ability to influence both the minds and the bodies of others, merely by making use of what Dr van Pelt calls 'this strange force that lies latent within mankind'. He published a book *Hypnosis and the Power Within*.[1]

David Waxman's[2] book is a mine of information on the subject of hypnotism and we have relied on it throughout our studies.

Franz Anton Mesmer 1734–1815

Mesmer[3] is recognised as being the man who discovered the hypnotic state. Even today, two hundred years later, people are familiar with the term *mesmerised*. He was born in the small village of Iznang, near Lake Constance in Switzerland. He first trained for the priesthood, but then changed his vocation and studied law. Later, at the age of 32, he obtained his degree in medicine. Mesmer combined earlier healing theories with the latest scientific methods of the day. He claimed that magnetic forces could be harnessed to restore the balance of bodily functions and relieve suffering. He believed the balance of "ethereal fluid", which was essential for health, was influenced by heavenly bodies. This fluid could be controlled and guided through the patient by means of magnetised iron plates, shaped to fit various parts of the body. Mesmer eventually found magnets to be unnecessary. He then believed that he could control the flow of this ethereal fluid with anything that he touched. We think he was developing the use of the power of suggestion. The results were often dramatic and surprising. Patients suffering from retention of urine, toothache, earache, depression, trances, temporary blindness and attacks of paralysis were cured. His reputation grew throughout Europe for years, until he was forced to leave Vienna by his medical colleagues. He moved to Paris and commenced a new practice, one of the most famous clinics in Europe, in which he treated every type of illness. His fame grew rapidly. Patients travelled from every part of Europe to attend his clinic. The consequence of this was that the medical profession became very hostile towards Mesmer. As a result, in 1784, King Louis XVI appointed a commission to investigate mesmerism. The commission failed to discover any concrete evidence of animal magnetism or of the invisible fluid. Consequently, Mesmer was struck off the medical register and the practice of animal magnetism was made illegal.

Case study of a blind woman

Mesmer's earlier clash with the medical hierarchy came when he treated Marie-Therese Paradis, the daughter of the secretary to the Arch Duchess of Austria. Marie, a brilliant pianist, had been treated by the medical experts unsuccessfully for blindness. Mesmer was consulted, his treatment was successful, and she regained her sight. Alas, at the same time she lost that sixth sense that made her musical expertise unique. Her parents became furious at her loss of income and withdrew Marie from Mesmer's treatment. Not surprisingly, she soon became "blind" again. His medical colleagues forced him to leave Vienna through jealousy.

James Braid 1795–1860

James Braid was responsible for the change of name from mesmerism to *hypnotism*. We assume this was to avoid the stigma attached to the name of Mesmer, which Braid found inhibited the use of this marvellous and potentially healing technique. Alas, even today, hypnotism retains a stigma as a result of centuries of misrepresentation of this valuable technique.

In 1841, a French magnetiser, Lafontaine, first interested James Braid in mesmerism. Braid said that there were no magnetic fluids involved in the production of the trance. He stated:

> "The phenomena were due to suggestion alone acting upon the subject, whose suggestibility had been artificially increased. This was easily achieved by fixing the patient's attention on an object."

Braid considered that there was no need for any of Mesmer's "theatrical paraphernalia", but one might say that Braid's method of asking the subject to concentrate on a shiny object was simply an alternative bit of paraphernalia. Undoubtedly, a certain amount of theatre can be useful in enhancing belief, but in most cases all that is needed is the reputation of the practitioner. Faith healing is a modern-day version of mesmerism. After much meditation, Braid stated:

> "There must be a physical cause, that a continued tiring of the sense of sight could paralyse optic-nerve centres, causing a condition not unlike sleep."

He maintained that the mesmeric state was, in fact, a form of sleep, and in 1843 published a book entitled, *Neurypnology, or the Rationale of Nervous Sleep Considered in Relation to Animal Magnetism.*[4]

James Esdaile[5]

In 1847, James Esdaile, a Scottish physician practising in Calcutta, India, in the 1840s, reported that he had performed 3,155 major operations using his own mesmeric technique instead of anaesthetic. This did not involve either verbal suggestion or eye contact. "I'm convinced ... that mesmerism, as practised by me, is a physical power exerted by one animal over another, under certain circumstances and conditions of their respective systems."[6]

Ambroise August Liebeault 1823–1904

In the year 1860, Dr Ambroise August Liebeault, a medical practitioner, founded a clinic at Nancy, France. He began to test the ideas of James Braid, using the method of fixed attention. He was the first to demonstrate the curative value of hypnosis on a large scale, for he treated thousands of patients in this way with outstanding success. Unfortunately, Professor Hippolyte-Marie Bernheim, a famous neurologist, tried to discredit him. Subsequently, however, after visiting his clinic, Bernheim was completely converted to Liebeault's views.[7]

Jean Martin Charcot 1825–93

In 1878, Charcot and his colleagues at the Salpetriere Hospital in Paris investigated patients suffering from epilepsy and hysteria using hypnosis. Charcot still believed in the use of magnets and the idea of magnetism in hypnosis. He stated that only patients suffering from hysteria could be hypnotised and that the hypnotic state itself is a form of hysteria. However, as a result of his findings, there followed a struggle between the rival schools of Charcot and Bernheim. Eventually, the views of the Bernheim school prevailed. Charcot and his followers were exposed as unscientific, and hypnosis came to be considered as a normal manifestation.

Charcot discovered, through the use of hypnosis, the true nature of hysterical illness. Up to that time it had been commonly believed that hysteria occurred only in women, and that it was due to a misplacement of the womb. From the large number of patients that he investigated, Charcot showed that the condition could occur in either sex.[8–10]

Josef Breuer 1842–1925

Josef Breuer, one of Freud's colleagues, accidentally discovered that the root causes of "hysterical" symptoms were painful memories and suppressed emotions, buried beneath consciousness. These symptoms could be eliminated, or relieved, by encouraging the client to talk during hypnosis, to evoke release of the suppressed feelings, enabling the relief of symptoms. Prior to this it had been considered that a hypnotised person could not talk while in the trance state. We give the following case study, of the first person who spoke successfully in hypnosis.

Case study
Frauline Anna "O". This 21-year-old physically healthy young woman had a powerful intellect, penetrating intuition, great poetic and imaginative gifts and critical common sense. Freud thought that owing to this last quality she was completely impervious to suggestion. One of her character traits was sympathetic kindness. The element of sexuality was astonishingly undeveloped in her. Anna, bubbling over with intellectual vitality, led an extremely monotonous existence in her puritanically minded family. Her illness included paraphasia (difficulty with words), a convergent squint, severe disturbances of vision, paralysis (complete in the right upper and lower extremities, partial in the left upper extremity), paresis (slight paralysis) of the neck muscles and somnambulism (sleepwalking). When her much-loved father fell ill, Anna devoted herself to him until her health gave way. Then further symptoms became apparent: headaches, more paralysis and illusions (such as when the walls of the room seemed to be falling over).

Breuer started treatment. He recognised that two distinct states of consciousness were present in the client. In one, she recognised her surroundings, was melancholic and anxious, but relatively normal. In the other state, she hallucinated (she thought her hair and ribbons were black snakes), was 'naughty' (she threw cushions and tore buttons off with those fingers she could move) and had "absences" (in the middle of a sentence, she would stop for a short period, then carry on as normal).

Breuer, guessing correctly that something had offended her, obliged her to talk about it, which caused the inhibition that had made any kind of utterance impossible to disappear. This change coincided with a return of movement to the extremities of the left side of her body. Previously, she spoke several languages, but at this point in her illness she spoke only English, apparently, and without knowing she was doing so. When very anxious she became dumb, or spoke some French and Italian. Her father died, which produced an outburst of excitement followed by two days of profound stupor. Her field of vision reduced, and she was unable to recognise people.

Breuer was the only person she always recognised. She began writing again, but refused nourishment. Her condition worsened and she developed suicidal impulses. At this point, the essential features of the case included: (1) the increase and intensification of her 'absences' into her self-hypnosis which she used in the evening; (2) the effect of the products of her imagination as psychic stimuli; (3) the easing and removal of her state of stimulation when she gave utterance to them in her hypnosis. These features remained constant for eighteen months.

Throughout her illness her father's death was always clear in her mind, despite rapid and violent mood changes. She occasionally imagined she was living in the previous year, on exactly the same day. Another characteristic of this whole period was her telling of stories during the evening hypnosis. If, for any reason, she was unable to tell the story that she had devised the night before, she failed to calm down after the treatment. She then had to tell two stories the next day before she could relax.

Besides these phenomena there were psychological events – which had produced the illness – that had to be addressed. When these were brought to verbal utterance, the symptoms disappeared. Dr Breuer was greatly surprised when this happened for the first time, by chance.

During a period of extreme heat, the client found that she could not drink from a glass of water. She lived only on fruit, such as melons, so as to lessen her tormenting thirst. Eventually, during hypnosis she was able to express her anger, which she had felt some time before, when this symptom first appeared. She witnessed in her English lady's companion's room that the companion's dog had drunk water from a glass. The patient had said nothing, as she had wanted to be polite.

After giving further energetic expression to the anger she had held back, she asked for something to drink, drank a large quantity of water, woke from her hypnosis with a glass at her lips, and thereupon the disturbance vanished, never to return. Many of her other symptoms were talked away in this manner.

It was during this period that Anna "O" coined the phrase "the talking cure". Following a long and meticulous symptom-removal procedure, Anna left Vienna and travelled for a while, but it was a considerable time before she regained her mental balance entirely and Breuer could say that she enjoyed complete health.[11]

Sigmund Freud 1856–1939

In 1887, while visiting the clinic of Liebeault and Bernheim in Nancy, Freud observed that a suggestion to act in a given way given during hypnosis would often not be remembered by the patient upon awakening. The forgotten suggestion was nonetheless still carried out, but the subject would readily rationalise pseudo-reasons for his/her unconsciously motivated act. This finding gave Freud his first insight into the idea that beneath the conscious mind lay hidden unconscious agendas, which were the primary determinants of human behaviour.

Freud nearly succeeded in wiping out hypnosis, by abandoning the name *hypnosis* in favour of the terms *pressure technique* or *concentration method*. He explains his reasons for using different names for the hypnotic state:

> It seems to me, however, that if one can reckon, with such frequency, on finding oneself in an embarrassing situation through the use of a

particular word, one will be wise to avoid both the word and the embarrassment. When, therefore, my first attempt did not lead either to somnambulism or to a degree of hypnosis involving marked physical changes, I ostensibly dropped hypnosis, and only asked for "concentration"; and I ordered the patient to lie down and deliberately shut his eyes as a means of achieving this "concentration". It is possible that in this way I obtained, with only a slight effort, the deepest degree of hypnosis that could be reached in this particular case.[12]

Carl Jung 1875–1961

Jung was first a student of Freud, then his colleague in the psychoanalytic movement. Later, Jung differed with Freud on the weight given to the role of sex in human relationships and they parted company. It is often thought that Jung believed that hypnosis did not work. However, one of his case studies, clearly an example of self-hypnosis, illustrates his belief that hypnosis can be successful and also shows quite clearly why he abandoned hypnosis. He tells of a 58-year-old religious woman who had suffered painful paralysis of the left leg for seventeen years. Her story took a long time to relate and finally Jung interrupted her and said:

> "Well now we have no more time for so much talk I am now going to hypnotise you." I had scarcely said the words when she closed her eyes and fell into a profound trance without any hypnosis at all! She went on talking without pause, and related the most remarkable dreams – dreams that represented a fairly deep experience of the unconscious ... When the woman came to, she was giddy and confused. I said to her, "I am the doctor, and everything is all right." Whereupon she cried out, "But I am cured!" threw away her crutches, and was able to walk... In fact I had not the slightest idea what had happened. That was one of the experiences that prompted me to abandon hypnosis. I could not understand what had really happened, but the woman was in fact cured ... I counted on a relapse in twenty-four hours, at the latest. But her pains did not recur; in spite of my scepticism, I had to accept the fact of her cure.[13]

This is an excellent example of how easily a person can go into hypnosis and make profound changes without any long, elaborate or ritualistic induction. We accept that Jung thought that he was not using hypnosis, even though he said to the students that it was such a demonstration. He abandoned hypnosis at that time through confusion and embarrassment. Years later, Jung seemed to accept that it had been hypnosis. This is also for us a clear demonstration that those in great need, or having great faith in the hypnotherapists, can go into a deep hypnotic state instantaneously. This is one of the many abreactions that are a common experience for hypnotherapists.

Hypnosis had been kept alive only by stage entertainers and lay practitioners until the shortage of psychiatrists during World War One led to demands for a much quicker form of psychotherapy. Hypnotherapy was once again revived and used both for direct symptom removal and the remembering of repressed traumatic experiences causing war neuroses. The war showed how valuable hypnosis can be in effecting the relief of unacceptable symptoms though a "reliving", whilst in the hypnotic state, of the traumatic experience that originally produced them.[14]

Milton H Erickson 1901–1980

The most famous pioneer of this form of treatment was Milton H Erickson, probably the most famous American hypnotherapist. His therapeutic approach emphasises brevity, often focusing directly on the symptoms of his client. Often his client would remove the problem without any conscious understanding of the process. Erickson attempted to understand the person's emotions and experiences, then communicated with the client's subconscious to resolve the trauma and thereby relieve the symptoms.[15]

We have mentioned how Freud realised that he could achieve various levels of hypnosis in a patient without formally hypnotising them. Milton Erickson turned this concept into a fine art and could communicate or give suggestion to a person's subconscious mind and thereby achieve a hardly recognised trance state, known as a *hypnoidal state*, without any form of relaxation, deep or otherwise. Jay Haley in his book *Uncommon Therapy*, explains how Erickson used hypnosis on his own son Robert to relieve pain after an accident. Notice that in the following example there is no "trance induction" or "loss of consciousness".

> "Three-year old Robert fell down the back stairs, split his lip, and knocked an upper tooth back into the maxilla [jaw]. He was bleeding profusely and screaming loudly with pain and fright. His mother and

I went to his aid. A single glance of him lying on the ground screaming, his mouth bleeding profusely and blood splattered on the pavement, revealed that this was an emergency requiring prompt and adequate measures. No effort was made to pick him up. Instead, as he paused for breath for fresh screaming, I told him quickly, simply, sympathetically and emphatically, 'That hurts awful, Robert. That hurts terrible.' Right then, without any doubt, my son knew what I was talking about. He could agree with me and he knew that I was agreeing with him. Therefore, he could listen respectfully to me, because I had demonstrated that I understood the situation fully. In paediatric hypnotherapy, there is no more important problem than so speaking to the patient that he can agree with you and respect your intelligent grasp of the situation as he judges it, in terms of his own understanding. Then I told Robert, 'and it will keep right on hurting.' In this simple statement I named his own fear, confirmed his own judgement of the situation, demonstrated my good intelligent grasp of the entire matter and my entire agreement with him, since right then he could foresee only a lifetime of anguish and pain for himself. The next step for him and for me was to declare, as he took another breath, 'And you really wish it would stop hurting.' Again, we were in full agreement and he was ratified and even encouraged in this wish. And it was his wish, deriving entirely from within him and constituting his own urgent need. With the situation so defined, I could then offer a suggestion with some certainty of its acceptance. This suggestion was, 'Maybe it will stop hurting in a little while, in just a minute or two.' This was a suggestion in full accord with his own needs and wishes, and because it was qualified with a 'maybe it will,' it was not in contradiction with his own understandings of the situation. Thus he could accept the idea and initiate his responses to it. The next procedure, with Robert, was a recognition of the meaning of the injury to Robert himself – pain, loss of blood, body damage, a loss of the wholeness of his normal narcissistic self esteem, of his sense of physical goodness so vital in human living. Robert knew that he hurt, that he was a damaged person; he could see his blood upon the pavement, taste it in his mouth, and see it on his hands. And yet, like all other human beings, he too could desire narcissistic distinction in his misfortune, along with the desire, even more, for narcissistic comfort. Therefore Robert's attention was doubly directed to two vital issues of comprehensible importance to him by the simple statements, 'That's an awful lot of blood on the pavement. Is it good, red, strong blood? Look carefully, mother, and see. I think it is, but I want to be sure.' Thus there was an open and unafraid recognition, in another way, of values important to Robert. He needed to know that that his misfortune was catastrophic, in the eyes of others as well as his own, and he needed tangible proof that he himself could appreciate. By my declaring it to be 'an awful lot of blood,' Robert could again recognize the intelligent and competent appraisal of the situation in accordance with his own actually unformulated, but nevertheless real, needs.

"We qualified that favourable opinion, by stating that it would be better if we were to examine by looking at it against the white background of the bathroom sink. By this time Robert had ceased crying, and his pain and fright were no longer dominant factors. Instead he was interested and absorbed in the important problem of the quality of his blood. His mother picked him up and carried him to the bathroom, where water was poured over his face to see if the blood 'mixed properly with water' and gave it a 'proper pink color.' Then the redness was carefully checked and reconfirmed, following which the 'pinkness' was reconfirmed by washing him adequately, to Robert's intense satisfaction, since the blood was good, red, and strong and made water rightly pink. Then came the question of whether or not his mouth was 'bleeding right' and 'swelling right'. Close inspection, to Robert's complete satisfaction and relief, again disclosed that all developments were good and right and indicative of his essential and pleasing soundness in every way. Next came the question of suturing his lip. Since this could easily evoke a negative response, it was broached in a negative fashion to him, thereby precluding an initial negation by him, and at the same time raising a new and important issue. This was done by stating regretfully that, while he would have to have stitches taken in his lip, it was most doubtful if he could have as many stitches as he could count. In fact, it looked as if he could not even have ten stitches, and he could count to twenty. Regret was expressed that he could not have seventeen stitches, like his sister, Betty Alice, or twelve, like his brother, Allen; but comfort was offered in the statement, that he would have more stitches than his siblings Bert, Lance, or Carol. Thus the entire situation became transformed into one which he could share with his older siblings a common experience with a comforting sense of equality and even superiority. In this way he was enabled to face the question of surgery without fear or anxiety, but with hope of high accomplishment in co-operation with the surgeon and imbued with the desire to do well the task assigned him, namely, to 'be sure to count the stitches.' In this manner, no reassurances were needed, nor was there any need to offer further suggestions regarding freedom from pain."[16]

In our class discussions, this passage, read to students, evoked responses that were disapproving of Erickson's approach. The students felt that Robert should have been cuddled and cooed over with waves of sympathy. They did not agree with Erickson's empathy (i.e. identification with the child's feelings plus a demonstration to the child that someone understands those feelings). Studying his approach, we see that he first acknowledges the hurt, then the realisation that it will continue to hurt. This is followed by a wish for the hurt to stop, and then a suggestion is made that it might stop. Note he acknowledges uncertainty mixed with hope by his use of "maybe". Next comes recognition of the meaning of the injury to the child: pain, blood loss, body damage, loss of self-esteem. After this comes a recognition of the quantity of blood lost, with a distraction in the form of a question as to whether it is good strong blood, and a suggestion that this could be best investigated in the bathroom. The fact of lots of pink water suggests good strong blood. He then acknowledges the fear of stitches combined with the calming distraction of a comparison with others' stitches, ending with a task given for further distraction for the child.

This demonstration of empathy by Erickson was received with deep scepticism. Let us look at the difference between "empathy" and "sympathy". Sympathy is the declaration of a wish to comfort. We have learned to give sympathy with kisses and cuddles. While sympathy seems to be the obvious, "nice" thing to do, it does not reduce the anxieties following an incident such as Robert experienced. We can learn to give empathy but it is no mean feat. Sympathy still has its place but perhaps after empathy. Empathy, on the other hand, will achieve this goal and the use of empathy is one of the main reasons why Erickson became so successful in his unique way of working, although at first sight it may seem a rather uncaring approach. Sympathy has its place, but empathy is of overriding importance.

Neuro-Linguistic Programming

Neuro-Linguistic Programming (NLP) was derived from a number of different psychotherapeutic techniques. Principal among these was Dr Milton H Erickson's unique approach to hypnotherapy. Originally called "The Study of Subjective Reality", NLP was developed by John Grinder and Richard Bandler after their careful study of Erickson's work. Like Freud's psychoanalysis, it has become popular because the word *hypnosis* has been avoided. NLP practitioners concentrate on communicating on the unconscious level, focusing on body language, eye movements and posture to gain insight into their clients' unconscious traumas. They are less interested in conscious communication and what the client has to say, except with respect to their desires or dreams. Thus, by communicating at the unconscious level, they attempt to emulate Erickson and other experts in the hypnotherapeutic field.[17, 18]

So What is Hypnosis?

In truth no one knows, and, although some experts would argue with us, we would define hypnosis as a state of mind, enhanced through relaxation, in which the subconscious mind is able to communicate with the conscious mind. In this state we are able to free ourselves from social conditioning; limiting inhibitions and opinions taught to us by parents, teachers, priests, doctors and other people generally. Having lifted these false restrictions, people are able to explore the largely unused potential of their subconscious minds, enabling them to do things that previously they believed to be impossible.

Is hypnosis dangerous?

Under a properly trained hypnotherapist the hypnotic state is not dangerous, but poorly trained operators could have distressing effects on their clients. This, of course, is true of any counselling or therapeutic method.

Do People Lose Control in Hypnosis?

Contrary to popular belief, however deep people go into hypnosis, they remain in full control. A hypnotised person is awake, able to talk, say "no" and, if needed, get up and walk away. A hypnotist, however good, cannot make a person do anything that is against their moral, ethical or religious code. People often ask: if this is true, how do stage hypnotists get people to do all those silly things? Here, it is important to remember that the stage hypnotist always asks for volunteers, and by volunteering, the subject is giving permission for what takes place – bearing in mind, of course, that most volunteers by now have a good idea of what will happen. And, let's face it, the jokes do not seem to change much. Are there not, indeed, many television and stage shows that exploit people's willingness to do very silly things, even without hypnosis?

Who can be hypnotised?

It is generally considered that about 60 per cent of the population can be hypnotised. We, however, believe that everyone can be hypnotised *if they want or need to be*. Everyone naturally enters hypnosis countless times every day without realising it. This is known as *hypnoidal state*. Of course, not everyone wants to be hypnotised, or is convinced of the competence of the researcher or therapist trying to hypnotise them. The researcher William Kroger states:

> Our lives are full of hypnoidal contacts and relationships, that are referred to by psychologists as "waking hypnosis".
>
> Repetitive radio and television commercials, advertising propaganda, and good orators or actors, heighten the attention span in a meaningful manner and enhance our suggestibility.
>
> When watching an interesting motion picture, our attention is focused on the screen, and we soon enter a hypnoidal state. Varying degrees of emotion are registered as we identify with the action in the film. Reality is made out of unreality. Whenever the necessity for reality is required, thinking is rendered unnecessary, a type of waking hypnosis occurs. After walking out of the theatre, we usually blink our eyes for a moment to orientate ourselves. Without realising it, we are in a hypnoidal state and on the way to being effectively "hypnotised". Waking hypnosis here occurs as the result of utilising ordinary experiences.[19]

The hypnoidal state is also known as *trance state*. Trance can be induced by separation from routine daily life, emotional tension, ambiguity and confusion, public confessions of feeling, listening to music, singing and dancing, fatigue, boredom, fasting and the use of caffeine, alcohol and other mind-altering chemicals. Professor John Shlien, Emeritus Professor of Chicago University, USA, states:

> These factors are all present to some extent in large group workshops, as well as in the course of psychotherapy, psychic experiences, healing, religious conversion, spirit possession, and many other activities. Persons in trance are able to extend their powers of physical agility and strength, concentration, perception, insight, and creativity, not only personally, but also to guide and maintain the collective.[20]

What are the limits of hypnosis or self-hypnosis

This book describes how hypnosis has been able to treat even the most advanced cancer. We also mention the positive effects hypnotherapy has had on genetically derived fish-scale skin disease and haemophilia, although medical science in general accepts that genetically determined conditions cannot be altered. As hypnosis is only communication with the deeper levels of the mind, it seems to us that the only limitation is that of the imagination. In other words, anything can be achieved, if one can imagine oneself being successful.

How does hypnosis relieve the terrible side effects of treatment of cancer?

There is now a general agreement among investigators of hypnosis that approximately 70 per cent of people with superior hypnotic ability can significantly reduce pain by at least 50 per cent. There is, however, still some disagreement as to whether hypnosis is a special state produced by a personal hypnotic ability and a procedure of induction, or essentially goal- or motivation-oriented – in other words, available to everyone if the need or desire is strong enough. Currently, experimental research suggests that hypnotic experience and behaviour are primarily dependent on individual ability or talent, and only secondarily on hypnotic procedure.

The significance of this is that any idea of hypnosis being produced by a power from the hypnotist has been discarded. Thus, hypnosis is something that comes from within us and is not an external force. We are of the opinion that there is no limit to the potential of the human mind once we can establish communication with the subconscious. Hypnosis is one of the ways that facilitate this.[21–25]

It was Theodore Barber[26] who suggested that hypnosis is essentially a goal- or motivation-oriented condition, the level of need being the most important factor. A client with a disabling illness will have a greater need than an experimental subject. He suggested that hypnosis is often a process of dehypnotising a person from a false idea or belief. For example, doctors tell us that we need medication to control pain, but Barber reported in 1977 that 99 per cent of patients could use hypnosis as the sole anaesthetic agent in undergoing dental operative procedures. Similarly, it is commonly held that we cannot control our blood flow, or heal ourselves of cancer. Nevertheless, a BBC television documentary,[27] in 1982, recorded a woman having a nose operation without anaesthetic and not spilling a drop of blood.

Examples of haemophiliacs controlling the flow of blood and people healing themselves of advanced cancers, just with hypnosis, are discussed in the next chapter. Obviously, these people have a strong need. All that has to be added is the right environment, in which the clients are encouraged to help themselves, and miracles *seem* to happen. We conclude, therefore, that it is not actually the hypnosis that removes the pain, sickness and other effects, associated with cancer. It does, however, facilitate the process of dehypnotising or deconditioning people from the false belief that they cannot control these effects with their minds.[28]

All this may sound very difficult – taking years of training – yet the case studies in this book show that at least it is not impossible. As for the difficulty, how can that be, when most of the hypnotic treatments reported in this book have happened by chance? Generally, when we are teaching people how to use self-hypnosis, it takes one weekend. A large part of this weekend is taken up by reassuring them that hypnosis is not evil and that it is impossible to make people do things they do not want to do, or make them reveal secrets against their will. And yes; absolutely everybody can do it – if they want to. Once the reservations have been removed, the actual process of hypnotising oneself is surprisingly simple; the more it is practised the better it becomes.

We see it as teaching people a new way of thinking. Often, society teaches us that we cannot do things. For example, we are taught that we cannot control pain. Yet most of us have seen a child fall and cut their leg, not even noticing until it has been pointed out to them, at which point they start to cry. We are also taught that we have poor memories and must repeat a passage many times before we can know it. Yet the ancient Greeks developed methods for remembering that show the opposite is true. These methods are called mnemonics. In the self-hypnosis class, our message is: yes, you can do it – *if* you stop being afraid, *if* you take the trouble to learn how to communicate effectively with your subconscious mind and *if* you can imagine that you will be successful.

Hypnosis has been particularly successful with children. This is probably because they have not been so conditioned into doubt and scepticism. Children are not so afraid, nor do they judge something as bad before they have understood it. Equally, they do not need scientific proof to tell them what can be done. They simply seem to listen, absorb and do.

Is hypnosis evil?

No! This idea is based on ignorance, and watching too many horror films. We believe that most religious practices use hypnotism to a greater or lesser extent – while denying it vigorously – when they use chanting (repetition), ritual (association), visual and auditory reinforcement of messages sometimes assisted by substance inhalation (incense burning) and elaborate dress by priests and shamans (Mesmer dressed up elaborately). Note Gindes's[29] formula for the hypnotic state, explained in Chapter 4: misdirected attention + belief + expectation + imagination = the hypnotic state. It is hard to imagine any religious practice without these items.

Is hypnosis present in counselling?

We would say that there is little difference between these two activities and that they can be used together. This answer would shock most counsellors and counselling or psychotherapy lecturers,[30] who, when quizzed, have no proper knowledge of hypnosis, but share the prejudices and reservations of the public.

Now that we have discarded any idea that hypnosis is a power produced from the hypnotist, another question can be asked. Are the conditions that enable a person to experience the hypnotic state, present in counselling? To answer this question it is necessary to examine the conditions that are associated with hypnosis: (a) goal or motivation orientation, (b) lifting the limitations, restrictions and inhibitions, (c) dehypnotising or changing a false idea, or belief a person may have about themselves and (d) right-brain functioning, such as creativity, ego integration, problem solving, emotional states, self-healing and relaxation. Are any of the above states present in counselling situations? All the above terms are associated with counselling. Ian Wickramasekera,[31] professor of psychiatry and behavioural sciences in Virginia, states:

> The clinical situation (doctor–patient) reactivates the dependency of the original parent–child relationship (transference). This increases the probability of regression into dependency and enhanced vulnerability to social influence and learning. The "core conditions", outlined by Rogers,[32] of empathy, warmth, positive unconditional regard and so on, are probably pure forms of the ideal parent–child relationship. If the patient perceives accurate empathy, warmth, positive unconditional regard, and so on in the therapist, his level of scepticism and suspicion in the relationship will be inhibited and his/her hypnotic susceptibility will be increased at least modestly (2–3 points or more on the Harvard hypnotisability scale).

In short, we see in successful hypnotherapy that the following factors are necessary: need, warmth, trust and imagination. These are also what one needs for successful psychotherapy or counselling.

A M Weitzenhoffer,[33] in 1957, also points out that Freud and most orthodox psychoanalysts have stated that hypnosis is a transference manifestation. It can be concluded from this that any procedure that intensifies the positive transference would increase hypnotic susceptibility. Weitzenhoffer quotes Freud as saying, "What he [Bernheim] called suggestibility, is nothing other than the tendency to transference ... We have to admit that we have only abandoned hypnosis in our methods, to discover suggestion again in the shape of transference."[34]

It is worth noting that different authorities have described over twenty stages of hypnosis. In clinical practice, however, these are reduced to four: Light, medium-depth, deep and somnambulistic. Of these four, it is arguably the light stage that is the most likely to occur in a normal counselling situation.

There exists, however, another stage of hypnosis that comes before the light stage, known as the hypnoid state. Through fixation of attention, for example, the monotonous stimulus of a white line of a highway induces a tiring effect upon the driver. This eventually leads to some degree of dissociation that can produce a hypnoidal effect, and this, in turn, can merge with true sleep, which, depending upon the degree of dissociation, resembles hypnosis. The hypnosis is characterised by some detachment, as well as by physical and mental relaxation. The attention span fluctuates more towards abstractional states, a sort of daydreaming. Since critical thinking is reduced, enhanced suggestibility results.[35]

Altered states of consciousness

When reading literature on counselling or psychotherapy, it is rare to come across the term *hypnosis*. However, the term *altered state of consciousness* does appear occasionally. Dr Carl Rogers[36] explains his impression of this state:

> When I am at my best, as a group facilitator or a therapist, I find that when I am closest to my inner, intuitive self, when I am somehow in touch with the unknown in me, then perhaps I am in a slightly altered state of consciousness. Then, whatever I do seems to be full of healing. Then simply my presence is releasing and helpful. There is nothing I can do to force this experience, but when I can relax and be close to the transcendental core of me, then I may behave in strange and impulsive ways in the relationship, ways which I cannot justify rationally, which have nothing to do with my thought process. But these strange behaviours, turn out to be right, in some odd way. At those moments it seems my inner spirit has reached out and touched the inner spirit of the other ... and yet with that extraordinary sense of oneness, the separateness of each person present has never been more preserved.

Ila Prigogine,[37] the Nobel prizewinning chemist, who Rogers mentions in the same paper, offers a different perspective. Briefly, he considers that the more complex the structure – whether a chemical or a human – the more energy it expends to maintain that complexity. For example, the human brain, with only 2 per cent body weight, uses 20 per cent of the available oxygen! Such a system is unstable, has fluctuations or "perturbations", as he calls them. As these fluctuations increase, they are amplified by the system's many connections, and thus drive it – whether chemical compound or human individual – into a new, altered state, more ordered and coherent than before. This new state has still greater complexity, and hence even more potential for creating change.

For 250 years this fascinating and valuable knowledge about the power of the human brain and how to harness it for powerful healing has been obscured. Why? we ask. Fear, prejudice, jealousy and lack of understanding are obvious reasons. Unfortunately, the theme is so rich in drama that it his been central to plays, stories and myths; and the imaginative exploitation of the fear element has contributed largely to its obscurity. We see hypnotism in a disguised form in various counselling modalities, although this might be denied.

Behavioural Counselling

John Watson[38] is said to be the father of behaviourism. He saw human beings as animals who have been "conditioned" – that is, trained – into our various forms of behaviour. It follows from this theory that unacceptable behaviour patterns can be eliminated by a process of "deconditioning", while more desirable behaviour patterns are installed by further conditioning. This reprogramming (to use a computer analogy) largely ignores the emotional aspects of the human psyche. This led the behaviourists to consider that it is not necessary to understand the history of a person who has a problem: they believe it is necessary only to teach a better way of dealing with the difficulty. However, this position has been modified in later years, so that emotional factors are taken into account.

Ivan Pavlov

As a result of Ivan Pavlov's experiments on the conditioning of dogs, the ideas of learning theory were developed. Hypnosis facilitates learning. Pavlov considered that undesirable behaviour is a learned response. The process by means of which such behaviour can be learned or unlearned is included under the principle of learning theory. Pavlov considered that hypnosis was a conditioned response to suggestions given by the therapist.[39]

Joseph Wolpe

In 1958, Joseph Wolpe[40] incorporated Pavlov's ideas of hypnosis with the work of Watson into a treatment known as *desensitisation*. There are two main methods used in therapy, *overt* and *covert*. Overt techniques deal directly with the person physically in the environment of their phobia. Covert techniques rely on mental imagery, there is no need for the client to be physically in the situation of their fear. Hypnosis has been used mostly with covert techniques.

Overt systematic desensitisation
Overt systematic desensitisation is the procedure most often associated with behaviour modification, in particular with phobias. The procedure consists of gradually exposing the subject to a real situation or object that he/she fears. Gradual exposure alone, however, is not enough. A response incompatible with fear or anxiety must also be present to counteract the fear.

There are four basic states considered to be incompatible with fear or anxiety: hunger, thirst, sexual arousal and relaxation. The most common form of incompatibility response used in desensitisation today is relaxation. Before approaching the feared object, the subject is run through previously taught relaxation exercises. However, hypnosis produces a greater state of relaxation than any other method. Once learned, it can be induced rapidly, thus having a great advantage over any other relaxation technique. See R I Atkinson.[41]

Covert desensitisation
In covert desensitisation the client, while in a relaxed state, imagines going through a carefully constructed fear hierarchy, rather than actually experiencing it. He/she is asked to signal by lifting a finger if a specific scenario proves disturbing. When this occurs, the images are immediately withdrawn and the relaxation is deepened.

Although some practitioners deny using hypnosis with this technique, it is probable that any form of deep relaxation produces a hypnotic state. The distressing scene is presented repeatedly in small doses until the patient can picture it without experiencing anxiety. Hypnosis, through suggestion, can provide one tremendous advantage in this technique. It greatly facilitates the production of imagery.

Humanistic Counselling

We feel that four principles are behind this general approach. First is that of holism, which we take to mean that we look at the whole person, including their environment. Second, we see that giving respect to the person and their intellect and understanding should always be present in our own attitude towards them. Third, we see what Carl Rogers calls "the actualising tendency within every human being, and that this means that everyone has the potential to be a successful and socially acceptable person. Fourth, we see that everyone has a basic need for a nurturing atmosphere for the development of their self-esteem, which is the basis of their self-confidence and potential for growth. There are a series of counselling modalities that come under this general heading, which include Gestalt, client-centred and transactional analysis.

Gestalt Counselling

Gestalt counselling depends largely on the awareness of the client's thoughts, body language and feelings, and the use of powerful imagery: letters written but not sent; the empty chair that the client is encouraged to fill with those they need to confront. Such exercises can help the client recall the past events, wherein they experienced damaging trauma. We can see the use of hypnosis in these imaging techniques.

Client-Centred Counselling

Client-centred counselling is based on the assumption that clients have the power to solve their own problems and to initiate growth, provided a nurturing and therapeutic atmosphere is created. The elements required to create this atmosphere are *unconditional positive regard, empathy* and *congruence*, which can be supplied by the therapist. The client-centred therapist asks no questions, does not analyse and gives no advice. Dr Carl Rogers, the founder of client-centred therapy, spoke of a similarity between his own and Milton H Erickson's therapeutic methods. In 1957, he made the following statement[42] "... I have discovered man to have characteristics ... descriptive, [of which] are such terms as positive, forward moving, constructive, realistic, trustworthy." Erickson held that "the therapeutic task is to arrange the conditions that encourage and facilitate the emergence of the unconscious as a positive force. People have, stored in their unconscious, all the resources necessary to transform their experience."

Rogers feels that this similarity of views, seeing the human organism as essentially positive in nature, is profoundly radical. Rogers believed in the capacity of the individual, in a growth-promoting environment, to move towards self-understanding and self-direction; and, looking at Erickson's work, he says:

> I find that he also seems to trust this directional aspect in the person ... Both of us have found that we can rely, in a very primary way, on the wisdom of the organism ... Erickson, although he worked in ways very different from my own, gave great importance to sensitive understanding. He believed that an attitude of empathy and respect on the part of the therapist, is crucial to ensure successful change.

Our research showed hypnosis to be present in people receiving client-centred counselling. During this research programme, sixty volunteers were taught how to use self-hypnosis. Their brainwaves were then measured while they were being counselled, hypnotised or acting as control subjects. Results showed that subjects receiving counselling had brainwave patterns the same as those in hypnosis, and different from those who acted as controls. These controls were subjects who were given a harmless pill as a placebo and basic relaxation.

All these points emphasise for us that hypnosis is part of our daily experiences without our knowing it in many cases. We further feel that, harnessed without fear and with care, hypnosis, hypnoidal states and hypnotherapy can be forces for growth and healing in a most valuable way.

Chapter 2

Hypnosis and Healing

Hypnosis is sometimes misunderstood and undervalued. Although many people believe that hypnosis can be used for stopping smoking, reducing weight and making people on stage look ridiculous, there is more to it than that. If we look a little deeper into the work of hypnotherapists, we see them helping people with depression, addictions and phobias. Hypnosis has been effectively treating people with serious illness for hundreds of years, but reports in medical journals have somehow been overlooked. Why should this be?

We believe that it is due to the fact that it has been against Western medical expectation. The conventional view has been that the mind has little or no effect on the immune system (the body's ability to protect itself from illness). We believe the exact opposite. We think the mind has a dramatic and far-reaching influence on the body.

Many people recognise that, when they are feeling low, they are more susceptible to "bugs" and illness. When folk retire without alternative plans, they often go into a decline or even die because they feel devalued and useless. Sometimes when a partner dies the spouse left behind dies of "a broken heart" shortly after. What do people feel on Monday morning? Not too energetic and sometimes ill. We all know the trick whereby a group of colleagues say to one of their number, "You're not looking too good today" or some similar remark. After the fourth mate has said this, the poor victim really is wondering what's wrong.

Paul Martin, in his book *The Sickening Mind*,[1] mentions that the number of deaths resulting from the shrapnel and physical damage of the actual explosions on the first day of a Scud missile attack on Israel, was zero. However, the actual death rate was 147 for the whole day, 58 more than statistics would predict. Perhaps death from anxiety? How does this happen? Undoubtedly, fear can kill.

We use the term "I nearly died of fright", but how do we protect ourselves from its actually happening?

Our immune system, we accept, is linked to our mind – every thought has a direct physiological result. Some of these effects we do not notice, some we do – when, for example, someone appears suddenly before us, without warning, and our heart leaps. How many death certificates state that fright was the cause of the demise? How many of the 147 deaths in Israel were so designated? They would be attributed to heart attack, stroke or lethal accident most likely. How often does this happen every day when some news item confronts our nervous system and precipitates a medical catastrophe, later labelled as above whereas it may be a post-traumatic reaction? Our immune system, at its best, depends on a healthy body and mind. How do we reduce our susceptibility to an overreaction to bad news?

First, perhaps, we should accept the possibility that our mental health may need a boost. Perhaps we could start with a more positive outlook on the future and the present. Whenever some new situation is presented and change is needed, either in the family or with colleagues, some of us react by counting all the negative things about it. Some of us will see all the immediate advantages. Many people live in a pessimistic aura, induced by a low self-esteem, so they cannot see any good things happening for them and, even if good things were to come about, they would not expect them to last. This outlook will disadvantage their immune system.

This chapter suggests an outlook that is advantageous and is dedicated to case studies and research demonstrating actual successful treatments of cancer with hypnosis, mostly after the person has been diagnosed as "terminal". We expect that there are many more cases that we were not able to find and very many more again that were never reported.

All the hypnotic methods described in this chapter are as effective today as the day they were written. This is even true of the last case study in this chapter, which was written over two hundred years ago. We believe that these treatments would be occurring daily, if it were not for the prejudice that has resulted in the lack of research.

E and A Green in their book *Beyond Biofeedback*[2] described our first case study. It shows a complete eradication of a terminal cancer with a remarkably simple hypnotic technique employed by Doctor H and a colleague. Doctor H, taking an opportunity to use hypnosis to control pain and blood flow, used hypnotherapy on a patient with bladder cancer. The cancer was originally thought to be operable, but preliminary surgery showed that it had spread throughout the whole body and the case was considered hopeless.

The man was sent to the cancer ward to await death. He was amenable to hypnosis and all suggestions for pain relief were effective, so Doctor H decided to suggest blood-flow control. While in hypnosis the patient was told that a control centre in the middle of the brain regulated all the blood vessels of the body. The patient was told to imagine the blood vessels as pipes. Could he do that? After a short time he said yes. Doctor H told the patient that one of the pipes controlled the blood flow to the cancer on the bladder and asked whether he could locate the pipe. The patient located that pipe and its control valve. Doctor H suggested that it would be beneficial to turn it off. This the patient did. The doctors decided not to discuss this event with their colleagues at that time, and especially not the ward doctor, who was against the idea of hypnosis for any purpose.

Their purpose in visiting the patient daily was ostensibly to control pain, but each day they hypnotised the patient and repeated their suggestions for blood-flow control as well as pain control. The bleeding was almost entirely stopped within a week, and the patient's appetite returned. After another week the patient said that he wanted to go home, and because he seemed so much better he was allowed to go home for two days. On his return, he said that the growth on the bladder, which he had described as being the size of a grapefruit, was now only the size of an orange. Eventually, he reported to the hospital only once a week, then had a month away. When the patient returned to the hospital the ward doctor made a cystoscopic examination of him and accidentally ruptured the wall of the cancerous tumour. He died of peritonitis within a few hours.

Autopsy showed that the cancer on the bladder had shrunk to the size of a golf ball and the secondary cancers had all disappeared.

Because of the unfortunate ending, this case did not reach the medical literature. A search of the literature showed not a single other example of this simple but seemingly effective cancer treatment. The cost of such a trial would be insignificant. No apparatus would be required. No drug costs would be needed. The only cost would be that of a daily one-hour session by a competent counsellor/hypnotherapist for a week or two, with possibly weekly one-hour follow-up sessions.

This method for treating cancer involves the use of hypnosis to control the flow of blood and bleeding. It might be difficult to believe that a person can control bleeding simply by entering the hypnotic state and receiving a suggestion. However, Dr Howard Miller explains:

> It was observed and noted, that the blood levels of various body hormones and chemicals were most significantly altered under hypnosis and post hypnotic suggestion. A marked reduction to normal limits was possible in cases of elevated cholesterol, steroids, blood sugar and catacholamines. It was also possible to maintain these at normal levels with hypnotic treatment. It was most significant to note also, that it was possible to raise and keep them there for various periods of time with post hypnotic suggestion. These alterations were accomplished without any change in diet, although once we were able to achieve normal levels, diet regulations were then introduced. Significant alterations of bleeding and clotting times were also observed to be capable of manipulation by hypnotic suggestion.[3]

A BBC television documentary entitled *Hypnosis: Can Your Mind Control Your Body?* (BBC2 copyright 1982 by Micheal Barnes)[4] discussed the work of Dr Kay Thompson on bleeding and blood clotting, in particular a case study of a haemophiliac (a person whose blood is unable to clot or coagulate, leading to excessive bleeding). The documentary showed this patient on a visit to the dentist, having had hypnotic therapy to control his bleeding. He had several teeth removed under hypnosis without the bleeding that would otherwise have been expected.

The documentary went on to explain that this instance is by no means unique and reported a medical study of two hundred haemophiliacs undergoing dental treatment. The control group, who had not been hypnotised, needed between five and thirty-five blood transfusions per patient. The ones who did have hypnosis needed only two or three.

Wallace La Baw, a researcher at the University of Colorado Medical Center, has reported that there is some evidence that spontaneous bleeding episodes of haemophiliacs may be precipitated by emotional factors. He also claimed that success achieved by some "preventive" measures may depend on psychic influences, especially if the patients treated acquire a new outlook on life. In spite of this, haematologists have given little emphasis to the psychological aspects of haemophilia. He continues: "The usefulness of suggestive therapy with bleeders has long been recognised."[5]

La Baw's group began with a six-month programme of weekly meetings with parents of afflicted children. This led to a three-month programme of weekly meetings of seven youngsters. This group learned to induce a trance state and an increase of relaxation with suggestions to reduce the severity of their condition. La Baw wants to encourage the use of self-hypnosis by these children more routinely than is usual, rather than reserve it only for urgent problems.

He offers three case studies to support his report. Here is one of them:

> A nineteen-year-old man – reported with the children, because he had been recruited to help in the programme – whose haemophilia was discovered when he was five months of age, has a similarly affected brother four years his senior. The patient had suffered multiple severe disabilities from his disease over the years. Biting his tongue once precipitated a seventeen-day hospitalisation. After using self-hypnosis, many weeks passed without his need for hospital. A coagulation time near normal was eventually obtained, the lowest in his record. This remission represented roughly an 800 per cent improvement over the five immediately previous levels.
>
> During a week in the hospital, other forms of treatment than transfusion, including suggestive therapy, were successful. Though bleeding tendencies are known to improve spontaneously, this patient's use of his suggestibility is thought to deserve part of the credit for his startling remission.

La Baw and his colleagues published the next case studies in *The American Journal of Clinical Hypnosis*[6] entitled "The Use of Self-hypnosis with Children with Cancer". An experiment was designed to help relieve the horrible side effects of the medical treatment of cancer for children, but also seems to have helped a few of the participants in other ways. Two examples given by La Baw are described below.

In a 24-month study, 27 young people aged four to twenty who were dying from malignant tumours were trained to use self-hypnosis to reduce fear, anxiety, depression, discomfort and anticipatory vomiting prior to medical treatment. This was a very successful method and all these traumatic and upsetting responses were diminished. We note that hypnosis was expected only to reduce side effects. We further noted the number of survivors and wondered whether the workers had asked themselves, after two years, whether the core illness had been affected. This article tells of eleven children in this study; at the end of two years, only three were still alive.

Case study 1

A seven-year-old boy with Wilm's tumour had had this condition for seven months and was surviving at the end of the two years. Anxiety, depression, insecurity and bad school behaviour led to his inclusion in the programme. After only two trance sessions, his hypnotherapist was enthusiastic about his improvement. The staff noticed aspects of progress as well. If given time to relax he could control anxiety and vomiting. He needed time, because he used self-hypnosis by going through a ritualistic induction procedure contrived by himself.

Case study 2

A girl of ten with acute lymphocytic leukaemia was included in the study, owing to her lack of cooperativeness during medical procedures. Her mother thought hypnosis was connected to the devil, so would allow her daughter to take part in only three trance sessions. Even within this limited time the child was able to relax and go to sleep more readily and was calmer during treatment.

The clinical procedure for the use of hypnosis by Wallace La Baw is described as follows:

The meeting place was a naturally well lit meeting room devoid of clinical trappings. The children sat in chairs of appropriate sizes in a semicircle round the therapist ... One therapist, more commonly the nurse, intoned the suggestive utterances, while the others participated with, or observed, the children ... The induction technique employed was the progressive body relaxation method, followed by restful psychic imagery of fantasised idyllic scenes common in the children's experiences, such as a tranquil mountain view ... The word sleep was avoided as children are particularly literal in the interpretation while in the trance state Following the induction of the initial trance state in the group, small talk in the group again ensued, ranging...on issues from, comment on the conjoint suggestive effort just finished, to totally unrelated topics of interest to the kids.

Jane Goldberg edited a comprehensive book entitled *Psychotherapeutic Treatment of Cancer Patients,*[7] in which she discusses the work of O Carl and Stephanie Mathews Simonton, who are oncologists and gives the following example:

Mrs G, a forty-five year old white female with inoperable carcinoma of the breast with metastasis [whereby the cancer spreads to other parts of the body] to the bone, was on a regimen of chemotherapy ... began psychological treatment when her cancer was first detected ... Through self-hypnosis and visualisation, her cancer was pictured as a soft sponge-like substance which was actively and aggressively destroyed by her white blood cells (men with large paddles beating the cancer to death), and her chemotherapy a strong poison ... Individual counselling brought attention to her childhood, which was marked by strong feelings of isolation, fear and despair, with psychological neglect by both parents ... The use of hypnosis was valuable in bolstering her confidence and self-esteem. Five months after treatment began, there were no signs of metastases to the bone, and the size of the mass in her breast was significantly reduced. In addition to her physical improvement Mrs G changed her behaviour in relationships by being more assertive and expressing more of her emotional needs.

Jane Goldberg describes the therapeutic method utilised for Mrs G:

Individual therapy is offered prior to the group therapy using a selection from the four following:

1. Ego strengthening (self-esteem enhancement).

2. Pain-reducing hypnotic suggestions.

3. Self-hypnosis.

4. Group therapy. Following individual work, this starts with a five-day retreat with a partner. Cohesiveness of the group and a sense of belonging reduces frustration, stress and loneliness. The group develops through two techniques:

   a. positive revivification: while in hypnosis clients relive certain events in their childhood both positive and negative, thereby relieving tension
   b. age progression: one benefit of this technique is the choice of meaningful goals.

The conclusion is that the patient's chance of survival and quality of life are improved with counselling and hypnotherapy. Mrs G was enabled to understand how her childhood traumas affected her adult life, self-respect and confidence, allowing her to change areas of dissatisfaction. The possibility of unconscious suicide (Freud may have called it the death wish) is shown in this case study. Happily, once the trauma of a depressive childhood was recognised for what it was and relieved by counselling, the medically impossible happened – Mrs G's immune system took over and regression of her cancer occurred.

Bruce Goldberg reviewed the Simontons' results in the magazine *Psychology: A Quarterly Journal of Human Behaviour* entitled "Treatment of Cancer Through Hypnosis".[8] The Simontons, authors of the best-selling book, *Getting Well Again*, report that of 159 stage-four terminal patients, 63 are still alive (20 have been lost to follow-up). Of these, 63 patients, 22 per cent are cancer free, 19 per cent are in partial remission, 27 per cent are stabilised, and 32 per cent report new tumour growth. In addition, 76 percent of these patients are maintaining a 75 per cent or better activity level in their daily lives. Here is another example of how terminal patients have, without surgery, chemotherapy or radiation (with their dire side effects), in 22 per cent of cases, been successfully treated and, in the rest of the group, 19 per cent–plus 27 per cent have had their death expectation halted or slowed significantly, with hope of a successful treatment.

The Simontons' treatment for cancer is described by them as follows:

The patients were asked to assume the stance that they would explore emotional factors as related to their health, with the possibility of altering the course of their malignancy ... A five to ten day psychotherapy session was conducted with each patient ... The number of patients per psychotherapy group ranged between four and eleven, with the average number being seven ... Each episode was coupled with mental imagery used for the purpose of desensitisation, addressing fears, adding flexibility to rigid thinking, and releasing anger and resentments. Other counselling processes were also employed. These included having the patient review early childhood decisions and improve emotional outlets through standard assertiveness training; goal setting; and a guided fantasy about disease recurrence and death, to clarify underlying beliefs and fears. The program also included education regarding the benefits of physical exercise, which helped the patient establish a regular exercise regime. Imagery drawings were routinely used as a projective tool to evaluate patients' and spouses' beliefs about cancer treatment and their own healing potential.

These statistics speak for themselves. The results of the Simontons' method of psychoneuroimmunology show clearly that patients who have this inexpensive treatment live longer. Here we have another use of hypnosis and counselling to slow and even bring into remission cancer for a significant proportion of severely ill patients – more successfully than the conventional medicine, which had given up on these patients and labelled them terminal. Hypnotherapy could be tried out systematically for a few tens of thousands of pounds. This would be especially valuable in developing countries.

V W Cangello in *The American Journal of Clinical Hypnosis*[9] presents an article entitled "Hypnosis for the Patient with Cancer". He begins with a statement that suggests that the situation is hopeless and that psychiatric treatment is not practical. He continues by saying that patients were unacceptable for their programme if their state of health left doubt as to the effect of hypnosis and the disease. Hypnosis was successful in the relief of pain and helped in the elevation of mood.

Dr Cangello's discussion of the 81 patients, of which 13 case studies were recorded, ignores case no. 11, concerning the successful treatment of leukaemia:

A 51-year-old female with leukaemia had had many hospital admissions of considerable length and was seen three weeks after a splenectomy [spleen removal] which had produced a dramatic remission of her disease. She had a very stormy postoperative course, complicated by wound infection. She was severely depressed and anorexic. A hypnotic induction was done using a disguised technique. Suggestions of good appetite and well-being were given. There was a dramatic improvement in her mental state and her appetite improved. She was discharged within two weeks. She was seen six months later and stated that she had noticed peculiar food desires for three months after her hospital discharge. At this time the patient was still enjoying a remission in her disease and looked and felt extremely well.

The hypnotic procedure for this research included a half-hour interview in which the patient's suggestibility, co-operation and mental ability were assessed. Hypnotic induction followed this and was reinforced as necessary during special hypnosis rounds or during daily rounds.

Bernauer W Newton PhD, in *The American Journal of Clinical Hypnosis,* presents an article entitled "The Use of Hypnosis in the Treatment of Cancer Patients".[10] For nearly eight years, cancer patients were treated at an outpatient facility (the Newton Center, Los Angeles, California) using hypnosis and psychotherapy. Basic concepts, assumption and procedures are presented and the issues and problems encountered are discussed.

Newton claims that a significant improvement in life quality was achieved, with two exceptions, in all those seen over three times. Here are his results:

Over eight years the Newton clinic saw over 283 cancer patients for at least one session. Age range 2–74 years: average age 44 years.

Adequate treatment 105 = minimum of ten one hour sessions over a three month period.

Inadequately treated 57 = Seen three times or more but less than ten; or, in the therapist's opinion, were trying to die with a minimum of discomfort.

Unknowns 121 = seen for less than three times.

Total 283

Newton goes on to say:

> Of ... 105 adequates, 54 were still alive and 48 dead, of the 57 inade-
> quately treated, 10 are alive. Among the adequately treated 24 either
> had no medical treatment or whose treatment had ... terminated six
> months before ... and still had an active disease process. Of these 24,
> 15 are alive and 9 are dead; three of those who are alive were
> involved in the program during the first two years. In addition, of the
> fifteen, nine have been pronounced to be in full remission, 3 ... stabi-
> lized, and 3 ... uncertain.

Newton's work is characterised by a first assumption that the most
important thing is to give the client a sense of involvement in their
treatment in a significant way. He emphasises the prime importance of the therapeutic process as opposed to visualisation.
Visualisation is helpful but not as important as the counselling.
This is in contrast to many programmes using hypnosis to relieve
side effects. In such programmes, the practitioners do not entertain
the possibility of cure and therefore ignore reports of cures. In the
therapeutic environment, Newton found that gentle nondirective
counselling was preferable.

Newton notes that a large segment of cancer-patient population
consists of individuals whose behaviour strongly suggests that
they truly do not want to live. Many times, this seems to be a reflec-
tion of their belief that they have no control over their lives.
Sometimes it is their reaction to a major emotional loss that has left
them emotionally bankrupt with nothing to live for. He recognises
two groups: one continues to believe that nothing can be done, the
other begins to experience some significant relief from discomfort,
which stays with them on that basis alone. They make it clear in
various ways that they are not fighting for their lives, but they live
much more fully and comfortably almost up to the moment of their
death.

Newton's hypnotic procedure included:

1. Visualisations of the immune system as a powerful healing
   force coupled with imagery of people bringing medical aid,
   destroying cancerous tumours and cells.

2. Achievements of aims and objectives important to the patient, stated on a hypnotic tape as if real, for home use, sometimes made to deal with specific symptoms.

3. Psychotherapy, explaining the concept that the patient, in dealing with their feelings, may be creating stress damaging their immune system.

4. Group therapy on a weekly basis, reducing loneliness and presenting an opportunity to share common experiences.

Dr Newton gradually changed his approach, giving more emphasis to an improvement in life quality. This reflected an awareness that unless life quality improved, many patients would not fight hard enough to overcome the cancer. However, his initial aim, to treat the cancer directly, had not changed.

T S Eliseo described his research in *The International Journal of Clinical and Experimental Hypnosis.*[11] He gave the following case study, of what, we would say, was an eradication of a fatal cancer, with hypnosis:

> A 50-year-old female had breast cancer with many bodily parts removed. When seen she was diagnosed as having metastatic intracranial malignancy (secondary cancers in her head) with intractable pain. She was distracted and disoriented to time and place, although aware of herself. When first seen she complained constantly of great pain throughout her body despite medication. The patient was seen three times for about forty-five minutes over five days. After the third session the patient discontinued the intramuscular medication, indicating that she no longer needed it. She continued the pain reliever, but decreased the dose to twice a day saying she felt fine and wished to return home. She was discharged. Follow up twelve months later found the patient had not been hospitalised and was living at home. This poor woman seems to be a patient in the last stages of dying, with a cancer that had spread into her head with intractable pain. In the paper from which this case was taken, Dr Eliseo makes no claim for curing a cancer with hypnosis, only better orientation to time and place, less confusion, some pain relief and the ability to achieve some level of self-hypnosis. We see this cancer, as reported, as definitely terminal but seemingly arrested.

Eliseo described the following hypnotic procedure for this patient:

Hypnosis was induced ... During the first session the patient was asked to think back to a time when she was happy. She recalled an event in the early 1930s for which she could not give the exact date, when she lived near the seashore and enjoyed swimming a great deal. The suggestion was given that she should imagine herself walking out into the ocean up to her neck and experience the warmth of the water. This would relieve discomfort and result in her feeling at ease and content ... In the second session she was taught to utilise this procedure by herself, to achieve comfort and pain relief, whenever she wished. Since she was judged to be terminal, suggestions for relief of all pain where given. After the third session the patient could discontinue the intramuscular medication, stating that she no longer needed it ... The patient was discharged. Follow-up twelve months later indicated that the patient had not been re-hospitalised and was living at home.

C G Margolis had his research published in *The American Journal of Clinical Hypnosis*.[12] He offers six cases of personalised hypnotic imagery, helping patients to reduce pain, improve mood, alter sensory experience and enhance coping skills. The article included a case study concerning a 27-year-old man familiar with the Simontons' work, who wanted to use hypnosis to reduce side effects of treatment and to increase his healing visualisations. He was soon using hypnosis on his own and after eight cycles of chemotherapy there was no more evidence of tumour. After six months there was no evidence of cancer.

The hypnotic techniques employed by Margolis were deep relaxation, ego strengthening (self-esteem enhancement), imagery and suggestions for changes in perception and awareness. The patient's visualised imagery was of firemen with hoses washing the cancer cells and chemotherapy down a gutter and a drain. This image was used twice a day.

Hypnotic imagery began between the second and third cycle of an eight-cycle treatment regimen and dealt only with his images of his immune system. The third cycle was his most discomforting. He vomited repeatedly for three days and was so nauseous and weak that his parents had to care for him for five days. The next images developed were designed to reduce these side effects of chemotherapy ... During his next treatment he was to remove himself from the procedures by putting himself in trance visiting a comfortable place.

Mystical mountain imagery was also used, which featured shifting sensory and visual events ... Vomiting and nausea lasted less than one day, he needed no assistance from parents and his sleep disturbances disappeared. Before his chemotherapy treatment was completed, he was using hypnotherapy on his own ... The remaining treatment cycles were handled with minimal discomfort – no more than a day, perhaps less, of nausea.

Dr H B Miller[13] had an article published in *Science Digest*. His work with cancer patients led him to suspect that malignancy is really a generalised disturbance, with the tumour itself being a localised manifestation. Two women, one with asthma and one with a duodenal ulcer, were given suggestions to encourage and enhance physical and emotional relaxation. Both women had associated breast tumours. The asthma patient had a malignant tumour, while the patient with the duodenal ulcer had a benign tumour. Both had refused surgery.

While under treatment for asthma and ulcer the breast tumours resolved significantly. The benign tumour disappeared, while the malignant one shrank to less than a quarter of its size. Suggestions were given to inspire calmness, confidence, a sense of security and, in addition, to increase healing power and rapid tissue repair. A determined effort was also made to guide the patient away from presenting fear to themselves. Treatments were continued twice a month for from four to six months, then once a month. After one and a half years, there was no sign of deterioration.

In the light of this experience, two cases of carcinoma of the cervix were accepted for treatment. Both patients had refused surgery. The suggestions given were the same as for the breast cases. Both resolved significantly. One progressed from a classification of malignant to a dyskaryosis (a borderline type). The other case regressed to a hyperactive, but negative, class. Both have remained in this state for a year, when reported in 1970.

Unfortunately, Miller did not report his hypnotic therapy method in this report. From the text, however, it seems clear that he used a series of suggestions directed towards a set of clear therapeutic objectives. These were first for relaxation, followed by one for increasing the patients' confidence in themselves and also a more positive suggestion for healing. This contrasts with hypnotherapy wherein associated counselling plus the suggestions helps a client to resolve past traumas that put a strain on their immune system. Two other cases had positive results.

The next five cases, of complete eradication of cancer, are all the work of one man, Dr Anslie Meares, an Australian psychiatrist. In *The Medical Journal of Australia*,[14] he describes the case of a single woman aged 49 with pathologically proven carcinomas of both breasts. She had had radical radiotherapy to both breasts, which led to regression of the tumours. However, they soon recurred with radiologically proven metastases. She underwent oophorectomy [removal of ovaries] but relapsed again and had treatment with Lactril, an extract of apricot kernels. Her condition deteriorated. She required a blood transfusion.

> When I first saw the patient, six months ago, she was frail, debilitated and in pain. Her left breast was wooden and immovable on the chest wall, the skin over it was so tight that it appeared in danger of rupture. The right breast had large wooden lumps in it and the nipple was retracted. Her general condition continued to deteriorate for the first six weeks in which I saw her.

Her weakness increased. She had severe pain in the back, and needed two more transfusions. She developed ascites (fluid in the abdominal cavity), which had to be tapped. Some weeks later, deterioration halted and she became stronger. Her abdomen, which required a second tapping, started to refill again, but drained itself. Three months previously she was able to keep down hardly any food. Meares reports that she was then able to enjoy steak and onions. Whereas initially she hardly had the strength to go for treatment, she was now swimming. The patient had no analgesic treatment during the later weeks. Her left breast was softening and was beginning to be moveable on the chest wall.

> The nipple on the right breast is no longer retracted and her abdomen is now soft to palpation. Her face has filled out, but there is still very marked loose flesh above and below the clavicles [collarbones]. In spite of the loss of fluid from her abdomen in the last seven weeks, she has gained nine pounds in weight. In six months, the patient has attended more than 100 sessions of intensive meditation, in a small group under my guidance.

The patient practised the meditation procedures, both in Meares's rooms and in her home. Meares had no doubts that her condition had undergone a dramatic change after meditation, not just for the relief of pain. "There is an improved attitude of mind, which one might expect from intensive meditation."

Meares's second successful treatment was also published in *The Medical Journal of Australia*.[15] He explains:

> I report a case of regression of carcinoma of the rectum after intensive meditation, in the absence of any medical treatment whatsoever. To date some 70 cancer patients have consulted me for 20 or more sessions of intensive meditation. The group includes people with various forms of cancer. In most cases the disease has been advanced and in some, truly terminal. Some few results seem to have been disappointing but some trends seem to be emerging.

He comes to the conclusion that the effects on the immune system of a profound and sustained reduction in anxiety are more important in this work than is the nature of the tumour itself.

> It may well be that the extreme reduction of anxiety in these patients, triggers off the same mechanism as that which becomes active in the rare spontaneous remissions. This would be consistent with the observation that spontaneous remissions are often associated with some kind of religious experience or profound psychological reaction.

A 64-year-old professional man consulted Meares. At the first meeting he was barely able to open his bowels and needed an enema each day. He frequently had to pass urine in the night. A biopsy showed that he had carcinoma of the rectum. The patient had refused an emergency operation. He instead asked Meares to treat him after hearing of one of his cures. He saw Meares daily and meditated at home one or two hours a day. Improvement was noticed after two weeks.

Four weeks later he no longer needed the enema and could pass pencil-like stools. After two months he was not only sleeping the night through but was confident he had beaten the cancer and went on holiday, where he was persuaded by a friend to consult an iridologist (a practitioner who claims to diagnose bodily aliments by examining the iris of the eye). The patient was upset by talk of prostate trouble and cancer and stopped meditating. He was advised to have immediate surgery and returned to Meares shaken. Following two weeks of Meares's treatment his strength returned. After twelve months he was passing normal stools and looked and felt well. He returned to his profession, except for three hours a day for meditation.

The third successful treatment was published in *The Journal of the American Society of Psychosomatic Dentistry and Medicine*:[16]

> The patient, aged 34 years ... on account of a large swelling on the left side of his neck ... had been told that with treatment he would have 2–3 months to live and without, 2–3 weeks ... Treatment by meditation was complicated by lack of co-operation by the Oncology Clinic ... Encouraged by the clinic he had been drinking quite heavily. He was actually encouraged by the clinic, apparently in the belief, that if he had a very short time to live, he might as well do as he liked. Despite minor bouts of drinking he managed to master the meditative procedure ... He saw me daily, then less frequently and practised by himself at home. After seven months the mass ... showed little change but his physical strength was well maintained ... he was told that the tumour in his neck could well press on his windpipe and so cause him to suffocate. The patient panicked at this suggestion and immediately sought physical treatment. He had a considerable amount of radiation and the swelling in his neck subsided. Now 2.5 years later, after first seeing me, he is still able to get about in reasonable comfort.

Our fourth treatment from Meares, appeared in *The Australian Family Physician*:

> The patient is a 54-year-old married woman, with two adult children, the proprietress of a fashion shop. Fourteen months prior to seeing me she developed a mass around her left nipple. She had a radical mastectomy four months after radiation from cobalt skin nodules and an ulcer appeared which did not respond to radiation. Tamoxifen was tried without effect and the patient was advised to have chemotherapy. She refused this advice as she had nursed her sister with cancer three years before she herself developed the disease ... The patient attended each weekday for a month, for intensive meditation. By this time there was clear evidence of healing. It was arranged that the patient should return to her home in another state and come back for treatment in a month's time. However, by then the ulcer had nearly healed. The patient said she was well and felt it was unnecessary to return for further treatment. She has ... however recently developed a bony metastasis for which she had cobalt radiation.[17]

The last example we have from Meares was reported in *The Medical Journal of Australia*:

> The patient, aged 25 underwent a mid-thigh amputation for osteogenic sarcoma [bone cancer] eleven months before he first came to see me 2.5 years ago. He had visible bony lumps of about 2 cm in diameter growing from the ribs, sternum, (breastbone) and the crest of the ilium (hip) and was coughing up small quantities of blood in which he said he could feel small spicules of bone. There were gross opacities in the x-ray films of his lungs. The patient had been told by a specialist that he had only two or three weeks to live, but in the virtue of his profession he was already well aware of his condition. Two and a half years later, he has moved to another state to resume his former occupation ... The patient has maintained a rigorous discipline of intensive meditation as described previously ... Since this report was written the patient has been declared free of active neoplastic disease.[18]

Meares explains how he prepares his patient for meditation:

> The preparation starts before the patient first sees me ... I also prepare myself for the patient .... My own genuine ease of mind is the most single important factor in preparing the patient for meditation ... The patient becomes secure with me ... I see each patient for two or three minutes before the session. A male patient takes off his jacket, loosens his tie and undoes the front of his shirt ... The patient must experience the communication by touch as something very natural, reassuring and helpful. The touch must never be tentative, or it will make the patient anxious ... I help the patient into the chair and help him loosen his clothes ... An anxious patient on his first session is usually reassured by my moving close to him ... Other patients, both men and women ... feel closeness as a threat. With such patients care is taken to avoid too close a personal contact on the first session ... My physical contact with the patient gives him to sense that the procedure is a shared experience.[19]

Historical Examples

James Esdaile, a Scottish surgeon, is responsible for the following example.[20] This doctor, aged 37 in 1845, was head of the native hospital at Hoogly in India. He performed his first surgery using "animal magnetism" as the only form of anaesthesia. He left India in 1851 credited with 261 major surgical procedures and thousands of minor ones.

Two hundred of these surgical procedures were for elephantiasis, which results in enlargements of the infected area and can involve scrotal tumours weighing from 4.5 to 47 kilograms (10 to 103 pounds). One contemporary observer placed the death rate for this operation at about 50 per cent. Esdaile's rate was between 5 per cent and 8 per cent.

The contrast between 50 per cent and 5–8 per cent is startling. Why no further research?

Dr John Elliotson[21] provides our second historical example. In the middle of the nineteenth century he suffered the same kind of uncompromising opposition as Mesmer (see Chapter 1), and was dismissed from a professional post at the University College Hospital, London because he gave public demonstrations of mesmerism. He was a firm champion of any cause in which he believed. Later, he was reinstated and invited to give the Harveian Oration. Elliotson had also been ridiculed by most of his colleagues because he pioneered the use in England of a piece of medical equipment that the majority of his contemporary medical practitioners considered to be gimmicky. This was the stethoscope.

Elliotson carried out hundreds of necessary limb amputations using hypnosis as the anaesthetic and no chemical anaesthesia at all. His critics said that his amputees were not hypnotised, but only pretending to feel no pain.

His case study is of a successful treatment of an advanced breast cancer. It was first published in a British medical journal called *The Zoist* in 1848 and was entitled "A Cure of a True Cancer of the Female Breast with Mesmerism [Hypnotism]".[22] This article caused considerable controversy within the medical profession at the time. This is clearly shown by a letter Elliotson received from a colleague that was also printed as an appendix in the same journal (see below). This startling case study, dating back 150 years, reported in the learned medical journal of the time, has prompted no subsequent research!

Elliotson writes:

On the six of March 1843 a person of middle height and age asked for my advice respecting a disease of her right breast. I found an intensely hard tumour in the centre of her breast, circumscribed, movable and about 5 or 6 inches in circumference; the part was drawn in and puckered, and upon it to the outer side of the nipple was a dry, rough, warty looking substance, of a dirty brown and greenish colour. She complained of a great tenderness in the tumour and the armpit when I applied my fingers, and said that she had sharp stabbing pains through the tumour during the day and was continually awakened by them in the night. She was single, lived with her mother and was a dressmaker to many ladies. I at once saw that it was a decided cancer in the stage termed scirrhus [hard cancer], and I so named it in my note book but did not mention its nature to her. I found on enquiry that in November 1841, having raised her right hand, she instantly felt a sudden and momentary violent, darting pain in the right breast. A week later she experienced it again. These dreadful dartings, to use her own words, began to take place a dozen times in rapid succession and every few hours. Her nights were disturbed; the dartings were always followed by pricking sensations and tenderness. The part now began to look drawn together and puckered and sometimes a little, to feel hot. Fomenting it with warm water gave relief but she discovered that it had grown hard. Her complexion and hands had gradually grown sallow. For many months she mentioned her complaint to her medical man Mr. Powell of Great Coram Street, Brunswick Square, but declined showing it to him, as he was a young man. The father's mother had died of a bleeding cancer of the breast. I proposed mesmerism to her. My purpose was to render her insensible to the pain of the surgical removal of the breast seeing no other chance for her; and this indeed was a poor chance, for cancer invariably returns in the same or some other part if the patient survives long enough; and the operation is not to be recommended unless it can be conducted without pain. When a disease termed cancer has not returned I have no doubt that it had not been cancer. Such a terrible thing as the removal of a breast, not cancerous, has always been, but too frequent among surgeons. Unwilling to make her unhappy, I said no more and allowed her to suppose that the mesmerism was intended to cure her disease. I mesmerised her for half an hour daily. Her eyes perfectly closed and she fell asleep near the expiration of the half-hour. At the end of the month her pain had lessened so that her nights became greatly better and her health and spirits improved. The sallowness of her complexion lessened. For the first six months the tumour increased and she could work no longer. She showed her breast, at her mother's request, to her medical man Mr Powell who immediately in her presence pronounced it to be a confirmed incurable cancer adding that if it were not cut away, it would be as big as his head by Christmas and that if mesmerism cured it he would believe anything. She thus learned the distressing truth, which I had so anxiously kept from her.

During Elliotson's occasional trips abroad he left her in the hands of a colleague to be mesmerised daily. The patient, Miss Barber, resisted many exhortations for surgical removal over some considerable time. The summer of 1844 passed on, the cancerous sallowness disappeared, she had less pain, her strength increased, and the warty-looking growth dropped off, leaving a sound smooth surface. And there was no increase in the diseased substance. A gland enlarged in the armpit during one of his visits abroad. Nevertheless, Elliotson began again and Barber slowly improved in every respect, and the mass began to diminish. The summer of 1845 arrived and a Dr Engledue examined her and pronounced the disease as cancer.

During the summer of 1846 the pain entirely ceased. During the year 1847 the disease steadily gave way. The mass had become not only much less, but detached from the ribs and moveable, again. The tumour continued to decrease, the tenderness eventually to wear off, and the gland in the armpit disappeared. The cancerous mass completely disappeared; the breast became perfectly flat and all the skin rather thicker and firmer than before the disease existed. Not the smallest lump was to be found, nor was there the slightest tenderness of the bosom or the armpit.

After the treatment of Barber, Elliotson received the following letter from John Ashburner:

> My dear Dr Elliotson,
>
> I have been today to see Miss Barber, your most interesting case of cancer of the right breast, cured by mesmerism. I cannot help sympathizing with you in your joyful gratification at this result, establishing your right to a victory over a disease that has always been deemed incurable. I pity the man who cannot rejoice in your success. Let the orators of the College of Physicians prattle in their pretty Latin, against mesmerism and mesmerists. Such cases as these form the best answer to their ignorance and folly, and establish the real dignity of the profession – a dignity for the maintenance of which the college was instituted, and the oath is administered to its members. You have vindicated that dignity by your labours in the case of mesmerism, and long may you enjoy the triumphant satisfaction which you must feel, mingled although it may be with melancholy at the stolidity, or something worse, of those physicians who refuse to assent to the truth, and who cannot respond to that eloquent appeal you addressed to them in your Harveian Oration. Let effeminate

minds throw their silly insults at you. It is but a paltry persecution levelled at a man of whom it will be said, as Charles Fox said on the analogous case of the persecution of Locke by the University of Oxford: they wronged a man "who is now their chiefest glory".

We see here several examples to support our case.

1. The bluntness of the patient's own doctor, who told her it was cancer, with frightening predictions and without any preparation. We hear so often, even today, of the bluntness and insensitivity of some medics when informing their patients of a dire condition.

2. Even Dr Elliotson was treating his patient to reduce her sensitivity to pain, assuming the need for surgery was ultimately inescapable; or, more likely, that she would die, and removal of pain without surgery would be the easiest way to die.

3. The patient regressed when Elliotson went on holiday, probably because the locum did not share Elliotson's faith and did not carry out his instructions. This underlines the need for rapport and empathy between client and practitioner and the value of emphasising positive aspects of the case. Elliotson saw no point in telling her that it was cancer and frightening her, with all the dreaded implications of that word. The effect of his positive attitude was a complete cure, although the original intention was for pain removal only. The openness of his mind distinguishes him from his colleagues and made the cure possible, for he could not miss the fact of remission of the cancer over and beyond the pain removal.

4. The description of the tumour's advanced state suggests the poor chance of survival, even given today's higher standard of medical treatment.

5. The locum GP's utter lack of faith in hypnotism. If, as some in the medical profession still believe, the mind has no serious effect on the immune system, how is it possible that this cancer went away?

The popular idea of the immune system is a series of mechanisms that attack an invading virus or bacteria. But the immune system is also active in eliminating any cell that is not under overall control of the body and in harmony with its needs.

This means that, if a cell turns cancerous, the immune system can recognise this and act to remove it. It is also thought that cancerous cells are induced daily in our bodies, by the action of carcinogens or by cosmic rays, which bathe us all, throughout our lives. The immune system functions to remove these cells daily, too. Our position is that a healthy immune system, doing this sort of job daily, can be overwhelmed by depression, fear, negativity, self-hatred and suppressed anger, which are, we consider, the most damaging forms of stress, often starting in childhood. These stresses can effectively remove the will to live. If, in the conscious mind, such stress can lead to suicide in the more usual form, then might they not lead to the less obvious unconscious suicide through a fatal illness?

Elliotson's treatment, although less flamboyant than that of the originator, Mesmer, was based on mesmerism, described by Pierre Janet in 1925. Janet tells us that Mesmer used apparatus of some elaboration and had a ceremony to accompany his 'hypnosis ' procedure like that at olden miracle shrines. His patients were taken to a hall with thickly curtained windows so that the ensuing rituals were in partial darkness. The music of violins filled the air.

The centre of the room was occupied by a large oaken tub famously referred to by Mesmer as the 'banquet'. The tub contained a mixture of water, powdered glass and iron filings. Its lid was pierced with holes through which iron rods emerged. Patients applied these rods to the parts of their bodies that were afflicted. Then they linked their hands and were expected to remain in absolute silence. Mesmer, seen as the "great magnetiser", would then join them holding an iron wand and dressed in a pale lilac, silken robe. He looked at all the patients directly in the eye as he passed along their rows, passing his hands over their bodies or touching them with the wand. Many were unable to feel any changes and said they felt the same. Others spat or coughed and some felt as if some insects were running over their skin. Some, mostly young women, would fall and go into a convulsive state, with coughing, laughter and occasionally delirium.

The hall was referred to as the Hall of Convulsions. The convulsive condition was called the "crisis" and was thought to be valuable. Then patients were carried to side rooms, where Mesmer's assistants would give further treatment. Two or three such sessions were usually enough for a cure.

Later, Mesmer maintained that he himself was the magnet and that no other aids were required and that the cures were due to "animal magnetism". When Mesmer made the passes a few inches from subjects' bodies, he believed that this invisible magnetic fluid flowed into their bodies from his fingers. He believed that this redistributed the energy and restored the balance. Having achieved this balance the patient was restored to health.[23]

We believe that the power of suggestion can assist people, in stimulating their own power to heal, which has often been severely inhibited by a variety of psychological blocks. These blocks are both cultural and individual. Hypnotic regression can more radically remove the inhibiting results of past traumas thereby amplifying the effect of suggestion. We see faith-healing, the placebo effect and meditation as having a similar effect on the human psyche. Sadly, sheer determination to fight is not enough, although it can have a delaying effect on the progress of cancer growth.

Chapter 3

Unconscious Retreat into Illness

The Death Wish

We feel the need here to comment on the death instinct (death wish or Thanatos) emphasised by Freud. This is the one theory that seemed never to be accepted by his followers. It seemed to them to be illogical, but it appears to us that many sufferers of serious illness find death a desirable alternative to their lives, which in some cases are too burdensome. It is also clear to us that counselling and hypnosis can enable a person to change their attitudes to their predicament and then find life more desirable. When this happens terminal illnesses are potentially curable.

Suicide by dramatic self-destruction is an obvious and regular occurrence in our society. The significant role of the Samaritans emphasises this point as well. Suicide by acceptance of an illness and subconsciously allowing it to become terminal is, we propose, a hidden form of self-destruction.

Dr Mark Schoen reports his work at the Cedars-Sinai Medical Center within a programme of psychoneuroimmunology in *The American Journal of Clinical Hypnosis*.[1] He studied patients with serious diseases, including cancer and heart disease, offering hypnotherapy to stimulate patients' immune systems. Schoen looks at people's "resistance to health". He says that patients "may use their symptoms to receive attention or avoid responsibility". This tendency will probably be hidden from their conscious mind and not recognised by them. It is seen in patients who deny the possibility that they are too frightened, depressed or tired of responsibilities to get well. In their unconscious mind a conflict exists, and their desire to become healthy is opposed by the gains offered by being ill.

He describes three themes, the first of which is *nurturance*. Here the patient receives attention and nurturance from others by being ill. Patients believe unconsciously that they can receive or justify this nurturance only if they are ill. This nurturance may come from family who give affection and attend emotionally. It can be from patients themselves, who have not made the time to slow down, and need the illness to justify the time needed to take care of their own needs. The threat of loss of nurturance creates this resistance to health.

This is illustrated by the following case study:

> Dr Mark Schoen gives an example of a forty-year-old woman with metastatic breast cancer. She recognised that her upbringing led to low self-esteem and a "caretaker" mode of life (looking after everyone except herself). She looked for approval from her mother and others, but, receiving little of this, became resentful. When she became ill with cancer, this unconscious resentment of having to attend to others' needs provided the very justification she needed to slow down and demand attention from her family. Once she became ill her family became extremely attentive to her. When the patient was asked, under hypnosis, about her willingness to recover she indicated that she was unwilling to do so.
>
> Through our sessions, her unconscious expressed and indicated by idiomatic signalling, a sense of safety and comfort in being heard and comforted in this direct manner. In this treatment the woman's unconscious experienced, for the first time, the idea that her needs could be met without being the family "caretaker" or needing to be ill. This experience enabled the patient to become unconsciously supportive of becoming well. The patient changed her mind and accepted radiation and chemotherapy and "has been in a state of remission for two years".
>
> The patient progressed from an unwillingness to become well (death wish), to an acceptance that there was no need for her resentful caretaker role, and an awareness of the validity of her needs, to have time for herself. Once this emotional shift had been made, her health improved through her desire to live.

Schoen's second theme he calls *withdrawal*. Individuals with setbacks in their lives will experience this. Such setbacks might be: bereavement, homelessness, large debts, loss of partner, redundancy or depression. All of which can lead to withdrawal and to illness. Let us look at another case study.

> A 44-year-old woman with bone marrow tumours suffered with rage, hurt and grief. She no longer had to focus on finding a new job or to re-experience hurt due to relationships with men. In the hypnotic state she expressed a resistance to becoming well. Becoming well meant dealing with a number of issues for which she was unprepared. She had pulled back from family and nearly all other aspects of life. The resistance to health was modified only after the patient became unconsciously assured that it was emotionally safe to get well. Because time was of the essence, hypnotic suggestions were made to create a distinction between getting well and having to deal with relationships and work. The patient then resumed her chemotherapy.

Schoen's third theme he calls *punishment*. This occurs when the patient feels the illness is deserved. This can be for having done something wrong or for having been a "bad" person. We illustrate this with a further case study.

> This is of a 24-year-old patient with cervical cancer. She attempted to please a dominating and demanding father by being a high achiever at athletics. Her failure led to tremendous rage, which she was unable to express to her father. So, instead, repressed it. This led to guilt and the rage directed at herself. In turn, this resulted in impaired self-concept, feelings of unworthiness and feeling of self-destruction. Her punishment had been, in effect, becoming involved in a relationship in which she felt totally unaccepted, and in a job were her employer was very demanding and critical. These were a reflection of her dynamics with her father.

> The patient continued a lifestyle that involved working twelve to fourteen hours a day, eating poorly and not receiving an adequate amount of sleep. When the patient was asked in a hypnotic state about becoming well, she stated that she was a bad person and that she deserved to be sick. The patient's unconscious was not willing to support health until she was convinced that she was deserving

of good health. Hypnosis was used to uncover the patient's rage at her father, and then to help her to express this in a direct manner, as opposed to directing it towards herself.

She learned that her rage was reasonable, and it was safe to express it with an acceptance of her feelings and an acknowledgment of herself as a person. This therapy led the patient to limit her work hours, improve her eating habits, take more rest and sleep, and terminate her destructive relationship. She agreed to surgery and chemotherapy and has been in remission for eighteen months.

A further example of resistance to health comes from Dr Frederick B Levenson's book, *The Causes and Prevention of Cancer*.[2] He gives an example of this in the following case study:

Karen was diagnosed by a cancer specialist as "hopeless" and given from three to six months to live. This 26-year-old patient, having had radiation, chemotherapy and radical surgery, was now in the last stages of deterioration: Emaciated, pale and physically too weak to walk unaided. Karen saw death as a separation from her children and sadness for them.

Levenson felt like crying and left feeling exhausted emotionally. His supervisor asked him whether he could treat this cancer or not. He was not sure, as it was so far advanced.

Karen's description of her wonderful husband seemed to suggest that she was treating him as she would a son rather than a husband. Karen's family, pious practising Catholics, had abandoned her when she married a Protestant. Although her parents felt guilty, Karen hated them for this and recognised that they had treated her as if she were a leper or had died. (Was she conforming to the role they had prescribed?) Karen's family were used to relationships with no affection. Karen described her mother as cold and unaffectionate.

Levenson began a long process of counselling with her. After several weeks, Karen's colouring changed from a greyish clammy hue to the paleness that many fair-skinned redheads or blonds have. When questioned, Karen acknowledged that she was eating more and not being sick. Levenson told her that she was looking much better. She immediately began to describe her never-ending pain. Levenson quickly added that it might not mean anything. Karen blushed and looked down in an almost coquettish manner. Levenson thought the blush came from Karen's feeling of being understood and realising her desire for love and affection.

Karen gained weight and passed the six-month survival limit predicted by the oncologist. Yonata Feldman, Levenson's supervisor, pointed out that the defence of self-destruction was no longer operating. No one had an adequate explanation, said Levenson. Karen, however, was telling Levenson, through her dreams and fantasies, of her sexual desires and the inhibitory Catholic upbringing that confused her. Her subconscious was rich with vivid imagery that portrayed her struggle against her death.

With hindsight, Levenson considered that the conditioned response of cancer had been extinguished. In the winter of the first year of her new life, Karen had become well enough to appear very attractive and began to have dreams that showed her sexual conflicts.

After the second year of Karen's treatment, the question arose as to why was the treatment continuing, when the original request had been to help the patient reduce her drug dependence. She was taking no drugs now. Karen now had no sign of cancer in her body. The process of her treatment seemed so natural that no one had questioned it until this point. The class, who were part of the supervising group process, seemed to think Levenson was responsible for her recovery. Levenson became emotionally involved in Karen's analysis and, instead of recognising Karen as a hypersensitive baby fearing annihilation through closeness to her analyst, saw Karen as an adult woman. He said, "In my ignorance, I was vulnerable. In hindsight it is all too clear what had happened. My lack of understanding helped lead to the inevitable premature end of Karen's treatment."

Karen started missing sessions. Several weeks later, she decided to end her analysis. Two years and ten months after the first meeting, Karen's treatment ended. As far as the medical experts were concerned, there was no sign of active cancer in her body. One month after treatment stopped, Karen was diagnosed as having widespread cancer. Four months later she died. "I believe that Karen died because I mistakenly put the baby down."

We perceive that Karen took the cancer path, rather than admit to herself that her husband and her relationship with him was unsatisfactory. Perhaps if Levenson had not felt rejection and consequently been in a different relationship with his patient, Karen may have been able to face the unthinkable and leave her husband. Even though Karen died, she had lived eighteen months longer than the maximum forecast.

As we read report after report in the scientific literature, of the effects of emotional state on physical health, we wonder why this treatment is not common practice. Below we show a few examples of articles we have read.

The first comes from Claus Bahne Bahnson PhD, reported in *The Journal of Psychosomatics*.[3] The article reports many cases of cancer following emotional upset. Bahnson is convinced that emotional upset causes cancer. He states that, for two hundred years, people have written that there is a relationship between cancer and stress. For example, Galen in the second century AD reported that melancholic women were more likely to develop breast cancer. In a further example, he quotes a report by Dr C Neumann, who observed that 80 per cent of her cancer patients had suffered the loss of a significant person within one or two years of the onset of symptoms. In 1979, Dr D Spence used a computer technique to count words referring to depression and hopelessness in a sample of patients who were to be screened for cervical cancer. Spence found that he could predict the outcome of the biopsy by the frequency of words reflecting depression and hopelessness. He blindly and by computer could pick out the cancer patients. Other researchers, working clinically with more than five hundred cancer patients, reached a similar conclusion.

The researchers Dr W A Green and associates, A H Schmale and H P Iker evaluated personality factors in patients with lymphomas, leukaemia and uterine cancer respectively. These investigators found that – in severe loss, separation with associated depression – helplessness and hopelessness are characteristics that signal the likelihood of the development of these malignancies.

Claus Bahne Bahnson explains that his own work resulted in an extension of the loss-depression theory in an attempt to detail why a loss should be more traumatic and crucial to cancer patients. In cancer patients the traumatic loss following separation during adulthood is associated with those who in childhood suffered disappointment, loss and despair with regard to parents. It seemed to be that people who developed cancer in adulthood were more likely to have suffered a traumatic loss following separation, through bereavement or divorce, during childhood.

C B Bahnson and his colleagues found that cancer patients indeed remember their parents as more neglecting and cold, as compared with other patients or normal control subjects. The parents are less loving, protective and rewarding, instead more rigid and stereotypical than are the parents of control subjects.

The next theme is family disintegration: Claus Bahne Bahnson observed that leukaemia and Hodgkin's disease develop, or worsen when the patient's family disintegrates. C B Thomas and her associates report that tumour patients rated lowest on the closeness-to-parents scale.

The next example is provided by Dr Daniel Goleman in his book, *Emotional Intelligence*.[4] He reported on a study of 569 patients with colorectal cancer, which showed that people who had said that in the previous ten years they had experienced 'on-the-job' stress were five and a half times more likely to have developed cancer, compared with those with no such stress in their lives. He found that weekly meetings for woman with breast cancer, in which they were able to express their feelings about their worries and their disease, led to a longer survival. On average they lived 37 months longer than their control group who lived only 19 months.

The researchers Schneck, Penn and De-Novo reported in *The Lancet*[5] that some people receiving kidney transplants developed brain tumours. Part of the treatment was the use of powerful immunosuppressant drugs to assist the body to accept the new kidney. When this medicine was discontinued the tumours were destroyed by the body. Immunosuppressant drugs work, as the word suggests, by suppressing the immune system, which is ever ready to eliminate foreign cells. While these drugs were present, the patient was prey to a host of diseases, including cancer. When the drugs were stopped the immune system came back to full effectiveness and wiped out the brain tumours. Similar findings were reported by Kersey and Spector[6] in their book entitled *Immune and Deficiency Diseases in Persons at High Risk of Cancer.*[6]

Daniel L Araoz EdD, a professor of mental-health counselling, reported in 1983 on some uses of hypnosis in *The Journal of Psychosocial Oncology.*[7] He wrote, "Most health care professionals are still convinced that hypnosis is more magical thinking than scientific intervention." He attributes the reasoning for this to the teaching that most medical students receive on hypnosis, most instruction being very brief and often very confusing. He explains that although the demonstrations of hypnosis are dramatic, they are not able to provide a scientific reasoning for these results and therefore the students do not understand precisely how it works.

He illustrates the value of hypnosis in the field of oncology for three areas: the control of pain, the control of other symptoms and the control of the negative psychological effects of cancer. One method for pain control is to suggest, under hypnosis, that a part of the body is becoming numb; another is to restore the feeling of chemical analgesia previously experienced. Further techniques involve disassociation from pain by using a goal-directed daydream, or modification of the painful stimuli by replacing it with a more tolerable sensation.

Hypnosis is also employed in oncology to reduce the side effects of any treatment, allowing the patient to continue with the therapy. An important point is made by Araoz in that hypnosis is often of benefit in providing an increased sense of self-control and self-esteem and helps patients to end their lives with a sense of inner peace and self-worth.

To us, there is no magic in hypnosis, or even surprise, when we read about a person living after receiving this treatment. We believe that hypnosis and counselling give release to the suppressed emotions of "I'm bad", "No one cares", "It's all my fault", "I should have said this", "I should have done that". Once these feelings have been discussed and understood, the person recognises that they are valuable, and that it was not all their fault. Their unconscious will to live (Eros in contrast to Thanatos or death wish in Freudian terms) returns, their immune system starts to work efficiently, and – hey presto! – they thrive. Yet this idea is still too radical!

The next line of Dr D L Araoz's research report is a direct denial of the evidence for the reduction of the size of a tumour using hypnosis. We would point out that both Bruce and Jane Goldberg, A Meares, B W Newton, Carl and Stephanie Simonton and others have reported remissions. The rest of the report, notes progress with hypnotherapy in the three areas mentioned, encouraging health-care professionals to explore the use of this technique with cancer patients.

Successes with Children

Hypnosis – and particularly *self*-hypnosis – has been successful with children. Once again, when attempts to control pain and other symptoms with hypnosis had eradicated the cancer, the results have been largely ignored.

A clinical report by Wallace La Baw (see p. 30), published in *The American Journal of Clinical Hypnosis*[8] discussed his work at The Children's Hospital in Denver. For 24 months, the study of 27 children and young people using hypnosis in combating some aspects of malignancies was recorded. The subjects, aged 4–20 yrs, were trained in group sessions to induce hypnosis in themselves. The gains from this were more rest, easier and longer sleep, more adequate food and fluid intake and retention, and greater tolerance for, and manageability during, diagnostic and therapeutic procedures.

"The focus of the initial meeting was to exchange information, establish rapport, set goals, and foster a realistic view of the usefulness of modern medical hypnosis," says the report. This is an example of an unrealistic but potent negation of the real power of hypnosis and psychotherapy in the reduction of a cancerous tumour. The group set out to use hypnosis only for the removal of sickness and pain and ignored or did not realise, its potential to succeed. One comment by La Baw was that some children were not able to put to work their suggestive capability, because they were boys and girls who needed to be very dependent on others. We feel that a remark such as this illustrates how many workers who use hypnosis have a diminished idea of its immense power. We believe it would be quite possible to work with these young people, first to reduce their dependency and then to enhance their individual independence and power to heal themselves.

The following three case studies are given by La Baw:

Case study 1
A boy of seven had Wilm's tumour for seven months. After surgery he was an anxious, depressed, insecure child whose obstreperous behaviour in school propelled him to La Baw's group. After two sessions his teacher was enthusiastic about his improvement. The child could control his anxiety and concomitant vomiting prior to treatment. He induced trance in himself through a procedure he himself contrived.

Case study 2
A girl of ten, referred because of her extreme uncooperativness, had had lymphocytic leukaemia for fifteen months. Her mother was very superstitious, through fears of the occult, and permitted her daughter only three hypnotic sessions. The enterprising child gained greater equanimity in clinical sessions and learned to relax sufficiently to go to sleep more readily. This patient was satisfactory, at the time of the report, written some time after La Baw's study.

Case study 3
A nineteen-year-old girl who had been wasting away with an osteosarcoma [bone cancer] for a year availed herself of instruction in our sessions in a nearly obsessive manner. She enthusiastically sought and gained control of her anorexia, anxiety and pain. She became able to take medication without nausea and vomiting, despite her previous general decline. She increased her appetite and converted her weight loss into a gain. This gave her time to achieve some personal goals. She dealt with her disease and her imminent death in a unique manner by speaking and writing publicly about her situation. Her record of reluctant dying garnered widespread notice, as she courageously succumbed at the halfway point in the study.

The idea of using self-hypnosis may be seen as less powerful than hetero-hypnosis with a therapist. However, research by John Ruch, which is significant in this context, is reported in *The International Journal of Clinical and Experimental Hypnosis*,[9] and showed that self-hypnosis is at least as beneficial as facilitated hypnosis. Ruch concludes:

> The traditional view, that a hypnotist is in control, has been gradually yielding to an increasing weight of evidence that self-hypnosis is the primary process and that the hypnotist facilitates the subject. The result of this study, by no means conclusive, simply suggests that this trend be pushed a bit further.

He proposes that self-hypnosis be recognised as the important factor and the hypnotist as the secondary one. Such a reconceptualisation is likely to be not only closer to current thinking, but also more accurate in fact, and more productive of further research.

Theodore J Jackobs MD and Edward Charles MA explained, in an article in *Psychosomatic Medicine*,[10] that over a two-year period 25 children with cancer were compared with a group of children without cancer. The families were questioned as to the occurrence of important life events of the parents, certain of which occurred with greater frequency in the cancer group during the year prior to the diagnosis. They presented the table of stressful life events shown on the following page.

A surprising 72 per cent of the families in the patient group had moved within two years of the onset of the illness. This compared with 24 per cent of families in the comparison group. The figures for moving for the one-year period prior to the apparent onset of the disease were 60 per cent and 12 per cent respectively.

This article quotes five case studies, the last of which tells of a fourteen-year-old girl whose parents were involved in an acrimonious divorce. In the course of this turmoil, the mother, with whom the girl lived, was forced to sell her suburban home and move into an apartment near the city. Initially, the youngster protested against this change and was extremely unhappy about it. Once the move was accomplished, however, the girl showed signs of adjusting to the new situation, but was very much troubled by the divorce and

Frequency of occurrence of individual life events

Life event	Patient group (cancer) (%)	Comparison group (%)
Marital separation	32	12
Death of close family member	20	4
Change in residence	72	24
Change in schools	56	32
Change in health or behaviour of a family member	60	24
Change in financial state	24	22
Personal injury or illness other than patient or control	32	12
Change in number of arguments with spouse	20	4
Major change in social activities	16	8
Wife beginning or stopping work	20	44
Son or daughter leaving home	12	20
Gain of new family member	4	12

Taken from Jackobs and Charles, 1980.

began to act out her conflicts by becoming hostile and rebellious towards both parents.

In this setting she developed a persistent sore throat, was taken to see a local physician and was found to have developed a premalignant lesion in the tonsil area. For some time thereafter, the girl's emotional trauma continued unabated, and six months later she came down with a severe case of mononucleosis (cancerous blood disorder).

We feel that in these types of cases, hypnotherapy could assist the child in coming to terms with the emotional distress, thus unburdening her immune system, which would then be better able to eliminate her cancer. Not only can hypnotherapy help psychologically, but also physiologically. It can give immediate relief while the longer process of therapy proceeds.

The following research illustrates this effect. Lonnie K Zeitzer MD and Samuel LeBaron PhD report, in *Behavioural Medicine Update*,[11] on the efficacy of hypnosis in reducing the side effects of chemotherapy in children with cancer. Chemotherapy-related nausea and vomiting are among the most aggressive of the side effects that cancer patients must encounter in battling with their disease. So severe are these side effects that carers have cited them as the primary reason for non-compliance by adolescent cancer patients, resulting in delay and even termination of treatment. Refusing or avoiding medicine was found in 33 per cent of one paediatric sample, and was as high as 59 per cent among adolescent patients.

In one study of chronically ill adolescents, those with cancer viewed treatment as worse than the disease itself. Fifty-four paediatric cancer patients aged between 5–17 yrs, some from the University of Texas Health Science Center in San Antonio, and the rest from the children's hospital of Los Angeles, comprised one study. Children were given hypnosis, non-hypnotic distraction/relaxation or a placebo (a sugar pill, as a control). Results showed that children in the hypnosis group reported the greatest reduction of both anticipatory and post-chemotherapy symptoms.

Children in the hypnosis group were given imagination-focused therapy. Initially, children were introduced to the idea of using their imagination while receiving their next chemotherapy course. During this session, which lasted fifteen to thirty minutes, the children were interviewed about their favourite games, television programmes, movies and activities. Discussion also included their pets, friends and family (to ascertain their names and what they enjoy doing together). The purpose of this discussion was so that the therapist could be most helpful in the shared development of a fantasy with the child. The therapist then helped the child to become involved in an imaginative fantasy. Following this experience, suggestions were given – both during and after the fantasy – for feeling "good" and for re-experiencing the same or other enjoyable and "fun" fantasies whenever the child wished. The therapist then told the child that he or she would be with the child during the next chemotherapy administration to enjoy a "fun imagination experience" and that the child might have some ideas about what they might "do" or where they might "go" together in fantasy during chemotherapy.

At the next chemotherapy clinic the therapist would spend five to fifteen minutes with the child to discuss the fantasy, before they entered the treatment room together (often with the parent) to become involved in an imaginative fantasy during the chemotherapy itself. During this fantasy, suggestions were given for security (e.g. holding or cuddling a pet), feeling good (e.g. being somewhere or doing something enjoyable), feeling hungry and wanting to socialise during the next few days.

There is now much research that shows conclusively the effectiveness of hypnosis in the removal of the side effects of the medical treatment of cancer, often described as worse than the disease itself. There is no logical reason why all cancer patients should not be offered this treatment. However, perhaps this caution is understandable, for the very idea that psychotherapy and hypnotherapy could treat cancer – yes cancer! – and not just the side effects is difficult to accept. Yet the question that must be asked is, since hypnosis is so effective in removing these horrendous side effects (which generally are difficult to relieve), why should it not treat the disease?

In an article in *The Lancet*, Dr Anslie Meares[12] wonders why a patient gets better although he, as a psychiatrist, has seen them only two or three times and has not made any direct suggestion of improvement. He says that he has nothing to give as an explanation, except a feeling that he has handled the patient well. He mentions the mind as being able to restore homeostasis (the previous healthy state) spontaneously in minor nervous upsets – a patient, ill for some time, experiences unexpected remission for no apparent reason. Colleagues confirm that this happens to their patients also. Meares asks, "Is it suggestion?" but observes that patients have been previously to other doctors, taken tranquillisers and received direct suggestion without improvement. Could it be that greater insight follows from the few talks?

But remission can follow the fewest words. Meares says:

> We know that nervous symptoms can subside after an abreaction. But this is not applicable because often-unaccountable improvements follow quiet interviews. Some patients have been ill for some time, and there is no reason why spontaneous remission should occur so frequently coinciding with their attending the doctor. Indirect suggestion is out, because so many have visited other doctors, had tranquillisers, or had direct suggestion from the attending doctor before, without improvement.

Overall, two features stand out:

> Several patients who appeared to have very complete insight into the
> psycho dynamics of their illness still retained their symptoms, but in
> each case my relationship with the patient was not satisfactory: On
> the other hand, several patients receiving insight therapy made
> apparently complete recoveries; but on looking back it seems that
> their degree of insight could not logically account for their recovery.
> With each of these patients I had a satisfactory deeper
> understanding.

Meares further wonders why, patients successfully treated by suggestion or "insight" psychotherapy, received very little verbal suggestion. He mentions that successful treatments were associated with a very positive relationship with the patient. He notes that successful treatments are linked not to the degree of training or knowledge, but to therapists with a high degree of empathy. He wonders why this seemingly illogical relief of symptoms occurs.

Meares does acknowledge that he himself felt calmer when in the company of a very calm yogi, and that this effect, of a person practising non-attachment (the absence of emotional reactions) was not an unknown phenomenon. Further examination of his and others' experiences leaves him still puzzled, and he finishes with a case study that he found baffling concerning a young, acutely distressed woman, who was much relieved after a consultation involving a minimum of talk and no drugs. After treating a patient for a colleague, Meares enjoyed the following telephone conversation:

COLLEAGUE: I have just seen the patient I sent you. She is really marvellous. She has not been as well as this for three or four years. I believe you fixed her without ECT.
MEARES: Yes.
COLLEAGUE: One of the new tranquillisers?
MEARES: No. I told her she need not take any drugs.
COLLEAGUE: She told you something she had kept from the other psychiatrists?
MEARES: No. She really told me very little.
COLLEAGUE: You hypnotised her?
MEARES: No. I could not hypnotise anyone as distressed and hostile as she was.

COLLEAGUE: What did you talk about?
MEARES: Really, I hardly talked to her at all.
COLLEAGUE: This is crazy. I'm going to stick to proper medicine. Anyhow, I'm glad you fixed her.

It seems that Meares has not read the accounts of Mesmer's cures. Mesmer often said nothing, just waved his hand and people were cured. It is not surprising that Meares has such success. Perhaps the faith people have, coupled with their own powers of healing (that Western medicine simply does not recognise) and Meares's own considerable calm and empathy, released their tension, and allowed their own innate recuperative abilities to operate.

Meares describes the nature of his meditation.[13] He distances it from classical meditation and the more modern visualisation meditation, and calls it "mental ataraxis". He then distances his method from hypnosis or autohypnosis (self-hypnosis). In reality, however, his meditation is a form of hypnosis as practised by Mesmer and Elliotson.[14] In the authoritative book, *Hartland's Medical and Dental Hypnosis*,[15] Meares's style of meditation is described as a form of hypnosis. Measurement of brainwaves with an electroencephalograph (EEG) suggests that there is no difference between meditation and hypnosis. Metabolic and EEG changes recorded during meditation have been reported in studies of yogis. The conclusion is that some forms of meditation bring about a state of consciousness similar to that found in a hypnotised subject. Work by Ananand *et al.*,[16] J P Banquet,[17] E I Rossi and D B Cheek[18] and J K Zeig[19] illustrate this aspect of consciousness.

Meares probably received the patient with a calm, friendly, empathic acceptance. Perhaps this was sufficient to create an atmosphere of trust, in which the actualising tendency (the ability of a human to grow and heal in a nurturing environment) could lead to healing. Although empathic acceptance may seem to be insufficient, it creates an environment of belief and expectation, as explained by Gindes's formula for the hypnotic state (see Chapter 4).

The immune system

Dr Howard R Hall wrote, in an article entitled "Hypnosis and the Immune System: A Review with Implications for Cancer and the Psychology of Healing", published in *The American Journal of Clinical Hypnosis*,[20] that the immune system operates to defend the body from bacteria, viruses and other pathogens. T-lymphocytes are responsible for the cell-mediated immune response. They protect the body from cancerous cells, which have molecular structures different from the normal cellular pattern. A cancer cell would be seen as different and be destroyed by T-cells. B-lymphocytes remain in the bone marrow and react to foreign substances, such as bacteria, by producing antibodies that circulate in the blood stream. Traditionally, the immune system is thought to operate independently of the mind. Some researchers have questioned this view and postulate the idea that psychological and emotional factors alter resistance to infection. Hypnosis may provide a means of examining this. Hall's report continues with some fifteen case studies illustrating the efficacy of hypnosis to improve the human immune response.

The first case study describes an eighteen-year-old girl having an allergic reaction to an egg-sensitisation injection. The reaction to the injection was a wheal (a slight swelling with reddening). On the following day the girl was deeply hypnotised and given the suggestion that there would be no reaction to the inoculation. The inoculation was given and no reaction occurred. On the day after that, the test was repeated without hypnosis, resulting again in the occurrence of a wheal.

The most dramatic is a case of Ichthyosiform Erythrodermia of Brocq (fish-scale disease), in which the sufferer's skin becomes thick and brittle, breaking with movement, and leaving wounds that heal only to break again. Although it has been seen as a genetic disease, it has been successfully treated by hypnosis in at least five cases. The dramatic effect of this cure is demonstrated very effectively in a television documentary on the subject. If one imagines the pain and discomfort of ever-breaking skin, the associated risk of infection and the immobilising effect this disease brings about, the amazement of those first witnessing such a cure is not surprising.

The first person to treat this disease with hypnosis was Dr Albert A Mason[21] (senior registrar), who was both an anaesthetist and a competent hypnotist. In a TV documentary,[22] Dr Albert A Mason said of "John", "The patient was a horrible sight. His whole body, apart from his face, neck and chest, was covered by a black substance that bore no resemblance to normal skin." Later, he wrote, "To the touch the skin felt as hard as a normal finger-nail, and was so inelastic that any attempt at bending resulted in a crack in the surface, which would then ooze blood-stained serum."

He mistakenly thought the patient's problem was thousands of warts covering the skin, and, after an unsuccessful attempt by a consultant surgeon to graft skin on a patient whose body was about 70–80 per cent affected by this black fish-scale condition, he volunteered to remove the supposed warts with hypnosis. This he did by suggesting to the patient that all the warts on his left arm would drop off, and then told him to come back a week later.

A week later, when the patient returned, the seemingly hundreds of warts on his arm had indeed gone and were replaced with normal skin. When Mason showed this arm to his senior colleague, the surgeon was shocked and said, "Good God, man, do you know what you have done?" He was given the name of the disease and told to go and look it up. Mason did so and to his astonishment discovered that he had successfully treated a genetic condition caused by the absence of oil-forming glands. Dead skin did not flake off, but built up on the body, turning black and inflexible, so that it continually cracked with movement.

Dr Mason continued to hypnotise the patient until almost all his body had been treated with similar success. Eventually, he reported improvements of 50 per cent on the patient's legs and feet, which previously had been completely and heavily covered, 95 per cent on the arms and complete clearing of the palms, although the fingers were not greatly improved. After three years this had remained stable. The consultant arranged for this case to be presented at the Royal Society of Medicine. This genetic disease has been successfully treated by hypnosis in at least five cases.

Further data supporting the contention that psychotherapy can be utilised to strengthen the immune system is found in Dr Daniel

Goleman's book *Emotional Intelligence,* which reports on Robert Ader, a psychologist in the School of Medicine and Dentistry, University of Rochester, who discovered that the immune system, like the brain, could learn. Ader's findings show one of the ways in which the central nervous system and the immune system communicate: through biological pathways that make the mind, the emotions and the body not separate but entwined. In his experiments, rats were given a medication that artificially suppressed disease-fighting T-cells. Each time they received the drug they were given saccharin-laced water. Later, Ader demonstrated that giving the rats saccharin-laced water alone suppressed the T-cell count, to the point of which some of the rats were getting sick and dying. Their immune system had learned to suppress T-cells, an impossibility according to the best scientific understanding.

The broad implications of this sort of work seem to be ignored. Western medicine as a whole prefers to hold on to the belief that the immune system is independent of thought. The general thesis of this book is that the mind has a significant effect on the immune system.

In an article entitled "The Treatment of Cancer Through Hypnosis" in *Psychology: A Quarterly Journal of Human Behaviour,*[23] Dr Bruce Goldberg wrote:

> The exorcism of disease-causing demons by shamans dates back at least 10,000 years and probably earlier. In the Chinese Nei Ching, the three-thousand-year-old Yellow Emperor's Classic of Internal Medicine, we are told amid discussion of acupuncture, herbal remedies and the physiology of vital organs, that the highest form of doctor uses no medicine, but treats disease solely through the agency of the mind. A prevailing view of cancer assumes that small microscopic tumours form in the body regularly.

Micro-tumours are produced continuously from the background radiation that bathes us all and natural carcinogens (cancer inducing chemicals) existing in the biosphere: smoke from fires, toxic chemicals from plants and man's industrial activities, and so on. These factors produce random genetic mutations, which can render a previously normal cell neoplastic (cancerous). This means that the cancer might keep growing until it kills you, without effective medication. In the person with an effective immune system, a defensive response is mounted against antigens (surface of an abnormal cell), and the budding cancer is destroyed by T-lymphocyte activated macrophages. If this immune response fails for any reason, the progeny of this one cell multiplies into a neoplastic clone and clinically manifests as the macroscopic tumour. This capacity of the immune system to monitor and control budding cancers is known as surveillance. The researchers recognise the need for further research and that cancer progression is influenced by psychological factors. This idea is discussed further in the following work.

James A Levenson and Claudia Bemis published in *Psychosomatics* an article entitled "The Role of Psychological Factors in Cancer Onset & and Progression".[24] Their article deals with stressful life events, and, in a section on metastatic and melanoma patients, they say both show longer survival times or more active coping if they have had some counselling. In a section on the immune system and cancer they set out to show that bereavement, stress and lack of social support can alter aspects of the immune system. For example, NK (natural killer) cells vary in activity with these factors. "Compared with other known risk factors, social factors may by themselves make a small contribution to cancer onset." This article is an improvement on those who would not acknowledge any significance but it ignores the work of Meares, the Simontons, Newton, and Jackobs and Charles's "life event table". We note the extreme caution with which many workers approach this subject.

Although Levenson and Bemis claim that the research method is flawed, because no controls are used, they do not acknowledge the dilemma researchers face when selecting those who will not be offered treatment. Do we just let them die without offering hope? One can see the type of control available when the outcomes of so many of, say, Meares's patients are so different from the clearly stated diagnoses of reputable oncologists. Much of the work cited in this book is with patients who had been given little time to live, after receiving all that Western medicine can give with startling results. It is true that Meares has not gathered people with the same diseases and treatment and left them to fend for themselves to prove a point.

Once again the researchers recognise the need for further research, but very little of this sort is initiated. We believe that one of the reasons why doctors are not offering hypnosis as a potential treatment for cancer is that they are afraid of offering false hope.

Meares states:

> In medicine we no longer expect to find a single cause for a disease; rather we expect to find a multiplicity of factors, organic and psychological. It is not suggested that psychological reactions, either psychosomatic or hysterical, are a direct cause of cancer. But it seems likely that reactions resembling those of psychosomatic illness and conversion hysteria, operate as causes of cancer, more so in some cases than in others, and that they operate in conjunction with the known chemical, viral, and radiational causes of the disease.

Despite the small but convincing evidence of the efficacy of hypnotherapy in the successful treatment (or remission in the cautious words of the oncologist) of cancer and the value in reducing the devastating side effects of radiation and chemotherapy, this treatment is rare.

We firmly believe that hypnotherapy, carried out by those convinced of its efficacy, as we are, could transform the treatment of cancer at a fraction of the ongoing costs to the health services.

Chapter 4

Only a Placebo Effect!

At one time or another, most complementary medicine has been said to be no better than a placebo – a "worthless" treatment such as a pill made of sugar. For many years, Victorian patients would be given a bottle of coloured sweet water because they seemed to be reassured with a bottle of "medicine" to take in their hand. It seems that this is still practised. However, on some occasions the placebo has been more effective than drugs, even curing an advanced cancer, as we show in the case of Krebiozen below.

The use of a placebo is standard practice in the testing of new drugs. One group of patients takes the drug being investigated, while another group receive a pill that looks the same, the placebo, and a third, the control group, receive nothing. The placebo always gets results, and the new medicine should be manufactured only if it attains better results than the placebo. As the placebo is only a trick, in theory it should achieve no results at all.

The power of the placebo should not be underestimated, however. We present a case history by S Kinklestein and M G Howard, called "Cancer Prevention – A Three Year Study" in the *American Journal of Clinical Hypnosis*[1] showing the placebo at work. It involved a controversial substance made from horse's blood, named Krebiozen. A terminally ill cancer patient heard that a new drug was being tested in the hospital where he was lying, not expecting to live. He begged for the new medication, and eventually he was given some. Ten days later there were no traces of the tumours, which had been as big as oranges. He was discharged. Two months later he was back in hospital, his faith shattered by unfavourable press reports of the drug, and his cancer reactivated. A doctor then gave him an injection of pure water, telling him it was a new type of double-strength Krebiozen, whereupon the patient recovered even more rapidly than before and again was discharged. Two months later he again learned that the American Medical

Association had declared Krebiozen to be worthless. Within two days of returning to hospital, he was dead.

The researcher, A K Shapiro,[2] says that a placebo is defined as "any therapeutic procedure (or that component of a therapeutic procedure) which is given deliberately to have an effect, or which unknowingly has an effect on a patient, symptom, disease, or syndrome but which is objectively without specific activity for the condition being treated". The placebo is also used to provide an adequate control in experimental studies. A placebo effect is defined as the changes produced by placebos. Another researcher, A Grunbaum,[3, 4] said that a therapy was a non-placebo, if it could be objectively proved that its effect on a disease depended on its characteristic factors; that is, if it operated according to the theory that described its activity. If a treatment has an effect that does not depend on the characteristic factors, but on other incidental factors, then the therapy should be called a placebo for these conditions. Grunbaum's definition calls for process rather than outcome studies, to show the non-placebo nature of a treatment.

As we have seen, the original placebo was a simple bottle of coloured water given to patients, to reassure them of their treatment by the doctor. It was not thought to be scientifically curative except in a minor reduction of anxiety.

An Example from Medical Trials

Here is an example of a placebo as used in medical trials. The researchers Lowinger and Dobie[5] tested the placebo response rate in four separate double-blind studies [where neither the doctors ordering the study nor the patients knew who received the drug and who received the placebo] between 1959 and 1962. The four studies were drug evaluations, each with a placebo control. The subjects of each study included 30 to 40 per cent schizophrenic patients, with the remainder being divided between those with personality disorders and psychoneurotics. The first study, in 1959, was a one-month evaluation of mephanoxalone, involving 17 drug subjects and 20 placebo cases. The placebo improvement rate was 24 per cent of the patients, while 30 per cent of the mephanoxalone patients responded.

The second study was initiated in 1959 and involved a double-blind comparison of amobarbital, captodiame hydrochloride and a placebo. At one month the 25 placebo patients showed a 74 per cent improvement, while the 20 captodiame hydrochloride subjects showed a 60 per cent improvement, and the 18 amobarbital patients were 78 per cent improved.

The third study, in 1960, compared trifluoperazine hydrochloride, chlordiazepoxide, meprobamate and a placebo in a double-blind design. Treatment continued from one to three months. There were 26 placebo, 22 trifluoperazine 4mg, 25 chlordiazepoxide 40mg and 21 meprobamate 1,600mg subjects. The results showed a 35 per cent placebo improvement rate in one month, while the trifluoperazine rate was 32 per cent, chlordiazepoxide 16 per cent and meprobomate 29 per cent.

The fourth study, which started in 1962, was a repetition of the third study, with double doses of the medication. In one month the 19 placebo subjects had an improvement rate of 76 per cent. The rate of the 15 trifluoperazine patients was 67 per cent; the 15 chlordiazepoxide subjects had a rate of 87 per cent, while the 16 meprobamate patients had a rate of 44 per cent.

Lowinger and Dobie[6, 7] then compared 15 different studies. Results showed significant therapeutic effects, ranging from 26 per cent to 58 per cent, with an average of 35 per cent. The conditions included wound pain, angina pectoris, headache, nausea, cough, seasickness, the common cold and anxiety. A similar variability in placebo response rate was seen, ranging from 24 per cent to 76 per cent in the studies on anxious psychiatric outpatients.

Lowinger and Dobie conclude:

> The implications of our results for drug evaluations become clear as we see the influence of the placebo response on the double-blind trial of a new drug. This points up a limitation of this technique upon which we have all grown dependent. The setting in which a new drug is evaluated is of considerable importance. For this reason it may be misleading to compare drug evaluations from different settings. The interaction between drugs and the environment in which they are administered is a continuing problem. The result of the present study may cast some light in this area, where drug proponents,

advocates of social psychiatry, and psychotherapeutic purists tilt at each other's windmills.

The placebo effect is not unique to just depression or psychiatric illness, but can also be observed in surgical procedures. Walter A Brown in *Scientific American*,[8] a researcher at the Brown University School of Medicine with a clinic in Rhode Island USA and a fellow of the American Psychiatric Association, has evaluated research of the placebo effect in surgery:

> Researchers led by Edmunds G. Dimond of the University of Kansas Medical Center in the late 1950s investigated the effectiveness of the then routine arterial ligation surgery to treat angina pectoris (chest pain caused by insufficient blood supply to the heart). The doctors performed the surgical procedure in one set of thirteen patients; with a second group of five patients, they made only a chest incision but did no further surgery. Among the patients who received the actual surgery, 76 percent improved. Notably, 100 percent of the placebo group got better. (Arterial ligation surgery is no longer performed.)

As well as in surgery, Brown describes research that shows placebo to be as effective as medication in regulating the heartbeat in patients who have suffered heart attack as well as in regulating asthma. Brown continues:

> The very effectiveness of a placebo is troublesome to us doctors and to other medial experts. It impugns the value of our most cherished remedies, it hampers the development of new therapeutics, and it threatens our livelihood ... Medicine has become vastly more scientific in the past century – gone are the potions, brews and bloodlettings of antiquity. Nevertheless, doctors and their patients continue to ascribe healing powers to pills and procedures that have no intrinsic therapeutic value.

Paul Martin in his book, *The Sickening Mind*,[9] states that placebo drugs and placebo medical procedures induce noticeable improvements in at least a third of all patients, often more. They have proved to be effective against a wide range of medical problems, including chronic pain, high blood pressure, angina, depression, schizophrenia and even cancer. He explains that the placebo effect is a significant demonstration of how our psychological expectations can override the signals coming from our bodies. Placebos work well if the patient believes in them. The effectiveness of a placebo drug or procedure is greatly improved if the doctor convinces the patient that the treatment will make them better, and if the placebo is administrated in a way that increases its psychological potency. For instance, placebos generally work better when injected, rather than taken as tablets. An injection has a bigger psychological impact than swallowing a pill. Pharmaceutical companies have discovered that, when a placebo is taken in tablet form, the colour, size and shape will have a bearing on its effectiveness. Those little pills may have to be pink rather than white.

A 1996 BBC television programme[10] investigating headache tablets showed that the placebo was 50 per cent effective. The actual medication was also only 50 per cent effective. However, the placebo did not cause a headache as the medication did.

Jane G Goldberg, in her book *Psychotherapeutic Treatment of Cancer Patients*,[11] explains how a doctor's attitude towards his patients can facilitate the placebo effect and healing. Goldberg describes the differing manner in which two doctors treat their post-operative patients. The first doctor is friendly to the patient and very positive about the results of the operation. This doctor then suggests some additional experimental treatment for the patient's condition: "You know it's a pretty benign treatment. There are some complications that could occur, but they aren't nearly as bad as the operation you have come through well …"

The second doctor is far more formal with the patient when suggesting the experimental treatment: "Now we really don't have any idea whether this treatment is any good or not, but there isn't much else we can do for you, so we would like to include you in this experiment. You may get the treatment or you may not, but if you'd like to join anyway you might get a chance at it, we'd be happy to have you. Before you sign, though, I have to tell you that you'll get sores on your arms and legs, you may get a fever or throw up, and you may get granulomatous hepatitis, or even anaphylaxis and die. But you'll probably be okay …"

Goldberg explains that the patients of the first doctor do far better than those of the second and believes the reason for this is the difference in the attitude they have towards their patients.

Placebo and Hypnosis

Is hypnosis a placebo effect?

The researchers C J Peek[12] and J D Frank[13] have studies to show the non-placebo nature of a treatment. Further research into pain control using hypnosis, compared with pain control with placebo, has shown consistently that hypnosis produces much longer actual pain reductions than those achieved with placebo. Further work by I Kirsh,[14] F J Evans and T H McGlasham,[15] M T Orme,[16] F J Evans,[17] N P Spanos *et al.*[18] support this demonstration. According to Professors E R and J R Hilgard,[19] induced pain reductions require high levels of dissociative capacity (the ability to fantasise), which are restricted to hypnotisable subjects. The same subjects are unlikely to dissociate following placebo administration, therefore, they show only small pain reductions.

Hypnosis and suggestion

Suggestibility has become an important part of research into the placebo effect and has been given as an explanation for the phenomenon. Although there has been some support for this theory, research into hypnotic susceptibility has shown this to be unreliable. We feel, however, that this area of research could be clarified if investigators first defined the difference between "suggestion" and "hypnotic suggestion". Bernheim in 1888 offered an in-depth formula for the workings of suggestion in the context of hypnosis. As a result, he made a very close parallel between these two. Bernheim viewed hypnosis as a state of enhanced suggestibility. This work is supported by other workers such as H J Sturpp *et al.*,[20] L White *et al.*,[21] H J Eysenck,[22] T H McGlasham,[23] M T Orme,[24] F J Evans *et al.*,[25] as well as H Bernheim.[26]

Currently, the trend to liken "hypnosis " to suggestibility is seen by some as oversimplistic. The close affiliation between suggestion and hypnosis has led to an abundance of tests that specifically measure hypnotic susceptibility. Further work by K S Bowers[27] and E R Hildegard[28] support these assertions. However, the researchers T X Barber and D S Calvery[29] have shown that responses to suggestibility tests vary enormously, depending upon whether the suggestions are introduced as a test of "gullibility" or "imagination". The fact that none of us would want to be thought gullible, but would like to be thought imaginative, may be a powerful motivational force.

Placebo and psychotherapy (counselling)

Psychotherapy is seen by some as purely a placebo effect. Simple faith on the part of the client that going to a therapist will help them. The attitude of the therapist towards the client, and not their skill and experience, seems to be the main determinant as to whether the therapy is successful. Further work demonstrating various aspects of the placebo effect is published by D Rosental and J D Framl,[30] N Plansky and J Kovnin,[31] N Q Brill and H W Storrow,[32] F W Hiller,[33] P Lowinger and S Dobie[34] and A P Goldstein[35] (consistent with C Rogers's view that the quality of the relationship between therapist and client determines the outcome of the therapy). This is widely associated with the acceptance of treatment and a successful outcome of the therapy. Cartwright in his 1958 paper, "Faith and Improvement in Psychotherapy",[36] states, "The term placebo effect could be replaced with patients' faith … It follows that, to establish the ineffectiveness of therapy, it would be sufficient to establish that the patients had no faith in it." He concludes: "… that therapists should stop worrying about 'placebo effect' and start conducting studies concerning actual functional relationships between different kinds of belief and improvement in psychotherapy."

L R Liberman and J T Dunlop,[37] in 1979, state:

> A logical complication of our concept of the placebo effect follows from the fact that some belief about the efficacy of a treatment is a part of any therapy. It is impossible to imagine a client who has no expectation concerning the psychotherapy he or she is about to undergo. The client's expectation is the result of many elements: the client's own history, his or her absorption of cultural lore about a therapy, what the therapist tells the client, and the therapist's attitude. Expectation surely accounts for an unknown amount of the success of any therapy. Increases in success should generate increases in expectation; the increased expectation may combine with the therapy, to produce even greater success, a spiral effect. On the other hand, research suggesting that the expectation is the only source of

improvement may reduce success rate and hence reduce expectation, a downward spiral.

They continue that it is impossible to have a placebo control group in therapy research, because the control group would have to have an equal expectation of success. Expectation, he explains, is a kind of belief; this he terms as the "placebo paradox".

What is the placebo presentation?

An examination of the available literature fails to provide a clear answer to this question. However, some familiar terms appear consistently: faith, belief, expectation, imagination. These terms bring to mind Bernard C Gindes's[38] original formula for the hypnotic state, which is: misdirected attention + belief + expectation = hypnotic state. We believe that most people are conditioned by Western society to rely psychologically on doctors and drugs, thereby inhibiting, very powerfully, their own natural powers for healing. We think that this sets the scene for the invocation of these powers when a placebo or hypnosis procedure is used.

Later, Waxman[39] explains, "… imagination is the integrating factor that welds belief and expectation into an irresistible force".

The only idea that appears in Bernard C Gindes's formula and not in the literature for placebo is that of "misdirected attention".

It was James Braid, in 1841, who developed the idea of asking people to fix their eyes upon a bright object to facilitate hypnosis. It was from this practice that the term "misdirected attention" originated. Previously, Mesmer's[40] technique of gently waving his hands over people had been used to treat thousands of patients with a vast variety of ailments. Bearing this in mind, and from our own experience, we believe that misdirected attention is unnecessary for producing the hypnotic state. We would replace this term in Grind's formula with the word "need". We have found that it is a client's *need* for relief of their problem, emotional or physical, that facilitates for them the hypnotic state. We also consider that it is the person's degree of need that makes the difference between high and low hypnotisability.

Let us look again at the terms for describing the placebo effect – faith, belief, expectation and imagination – and consider again Gindes's formula replacing the term "misdirected attention" with the term "need". Recalling the case study described on the first page of this chapter, with Krebiozen, it is clear how desperately the patient "needed" to believe in his medicine and how readily he accepted it. We would therefore surmise that the placebo effect is a form of hypnosis. We would further suggest that the placebo effect is a form of *self*-hypnosis. Self-hypnosis may seem unlikely to achieve the dramatic results described in relation to Krebiozen. However, John Ruch[41] showed that self-hypnosis was as effective, as facilitated hypnosis. J D Shea in his paper, "Suggestion, Placebo and Expectation",[42] concludes:

> This discussion has considered questions about the power of self-healing abilities that follow suggestion, and some of the personal strategies and personal qualities that might be useful to start self-change and self-healing. It seems a reasonable conclusion that placebo effects can be found in all types of illness and that these effects are often extraordinary. Greater changes in immune responses, where described in this paper, result from expectation of relaxation training rather than from the relaxation itself. A fascinating body of research suggests that psychological strategies, such as hypnosis, relaxation training, and meditation, may facilitate the development of changes in the system's readiness to focus on, and utilise, imagery for self-change and healing ...

Our own experience of training people in self-hypnosis or deep relaxation suggests that most people can acquire these skills sufficiently, to make a significant impact on their well-being. Thus, every person may be susceptible to suggestive modes of influence. It might also be remembered that hypnosis and other forms of altered attention, may be induced with or without going through a relaxation ritual.

The placebo effect is a form of self-hypnosis. We agree with Lowinger and Dobie, that it does seem impossible to imagine a client who has no expectation about the results of the therapy undertaken. Thus, the placebo effect must play a part in all psychotherapy and medicine. We also agree with Lowinger's research of the placebo response rate in drug evaluations, and indeed, the medication itself, upon which we have become dependent, is limited. Overall, we see these papers emphasising the point that for most physicians, the placebo effect is a puzzling anomaly, a mystery, which makes drug testing difficult, and is itself difficult to study. We ask them to see it as we see it: as the power that human beings have of treating themselves even for major diseases when they are in the right therapeutic environment.

Chapter 5

Why Me?

A Matter of Guilt

If people, through therapy, become aware that their cancer has been brought on by stress, would they feel guilty? Some may. Should they? Some doctors have not accepted our offer of free hypnotherapy for patients because of the negativity associated with this idea.

Who is to blame? Much cancer results from the stresses of life, which, finding no expression, are internalised destructively. Hypnotherapy is one way of relieving the effects of such stresses, freeing the immune system to deal with the cancer.

Who is to blame? No one and everyone. Where in the national curriculum do we learn to look after ourselves? Who taught the victim to internalise their stresses, and not discharge them harmlessly? How do we discharge stress? How much stress arises from our attitude to the stimuli that life has to offer?

An examination of the attitudes we carry shows a series of "shoulds", "musts" and "oughts", many of which are placed there by those no longer with us.

The Authors' Case Studies

We believe that to treat a cancer successfully rather than simply delay its course, the underlying cause must be discovered. We also hold that the cause, in part at least, is more often psychological than has been generally considered.

Our healing philosophy

Our beliefs can be summarised thus. We consider that a large number of illnesses have as their origin a kind of psychological content, which is hidden in the subconscious mind. In some cases the psychological trauma is not hidden but would seem to have nothing to do with the illness. The case studies in this book are related to cancer, but we consider that most illness has an element of this psychological content. The subconscious, according to common belief, is not only hidden but out of reach except by a psychoanalyst. Professor John Shlien,[1] however, considers that the subconscious has a series of levels of consciousness, with varying degrees of difficulty of access, but which can be accessed by oneself in the right circumstances.

We further believe that the immune system is not only there to fight germs, but is an elaborate repair system, able to seek out a tumour and destroy it completely. It can eradicate most illness if it is not preoccupied with psychological burdens. For many years it has been thought that it was an automatic system independent of the mind. However, we believe that the two are entwined. We further believe that psychological trauma can take away the will to live and the immune system dutifully follows, so we become vulnerable to illness. Such trauma could be for example:

- unhappy childhood
- bullying at school
- frustrated development
- overprotective loving parents (particularly in the teens)
- lack of satisfying employment
- unhappy marriage or end of relationship
- postnatal depression
- being overburdened with parental responsibilities (for instance, too many children, not enough funds, no partner, social isolation, empty-nest syndrome because children have left home, leaving the parent feeling redundant)
- job redundancy
- retirement
- fear of death

Bereavement at any age can be very detrimental to health and can take away the will to live. If with suitable therapy the effects of these traumas can be reduced, our will to live can be revived, and our immune system can set about curing even major illnesses.

The power to heal ourselves can be stimulated to such an extent that for instance we can control pain, control blood flow, increase the blood's clotting ability, overcome hormone deficiencies, reduce swelling and increase the rate of healing, reduce the severity of asthma attacks, reduce sensitivity to allergic materials and overcome addictions.

This power of self-healing can also be used to enhance mental and physical characteristics: for example, memory, strength, confidence, breast enlargement, easier childbirth, more control over our bodies and lives. Anything can be considered, even overcoming a genetic defect (discussed later) if success can be imagined and believed possible.

Our counselling philosophy

Our philosophy is based on the work of Carl Rogers and Milton H Erickson, whose underlying beliefs were similar, despite some considerable differences in technique. Rogers believed in what he called the "actualising tendency ", which is the innate potential of the individual to develop his or her full capabilities. The actualising tendency means that we have within ourselves all the resources we need to heal ourselves. This is most effective in a nurturing environment. Rogers believed such an atmosphere would comprise at least three elements: unconditional positive regard, empathy and congruence.

Method

Our first action with a new client is to outline our philosophy in simple terms, and here we are guided by an agreement reached with the client. We usually commence with an hour or so of client-centred counselling (nonhypnotic) (the essence of this approach is explained in Chapter 6 with the treatment of Dibs by Axline). The length of time, is variable and will be guided by the client's needs.

We then explain that the process of hypnosis involves collaboration with trust and not control. We make it clear that, should the hypnotist say or do something the client does not like, the client is perfectly able to say so and, if necessary, get up and leave. The client is then offered his or her first experience of entering hypnosis with relaxation and a few suggestions, and then coming out. If the client is willing and enthusiastic, we would then proceed to the next stage, which is hypnotic regression therapy wherein we invite them to recall a time and place in their life where some negative experience affected their health or happiness. This may refer to the earliest years of their life. Hypnosis can enhance their memory of such incidents.

After the client has recalled something of this nature, the next stage is to encourage them to review the experience and facilitate their examination of its consequences and effects. This process allows the client to make new choices as to their attitudes and behaviour in response to the trauma, and to draw conclusions about how previous choices have influenced their lives. At this stage they often experience a spontaneous rejection of the influences these earlier events and decisions have had on their lives. At other times rejection comes only after many sessions and many reviews.

The next, or parallel, process which seems appropriate, is the giving of direct suggestions for healing and enhancing the immune system, as well as suggestions for improving self-esteem and confidence in daily life. Often, in addition, clients will tell us what they want and make suggestions to be included in the therapy. We are happy to add these ideas for integration, either during hypnosis or outside the sessions. We also encourage people to enrol on a course of self-hypnosis, to enhance and, finally, take over the healing process for themselves. We believe that all hypnosis is really self-hypnosis.

Case study 1
"Why has this happened to me?" – Ms X a cancer patient.

History of presenting symptoms
Ms X was 27 years old when she discovered a lump in her left breast for which she was referred to a consultant at the Royal

Marsden Hospital, London, UK, where a biopsy was done. The consultant told her that the lump was a benign tumour, which required a small section of her breast to be removed to prevent it from becoming malignant. At this Ms X replied, "Why has this happened to me?" She was told "We do not know what causes it. We know it is not genetic, but it seems to run in families."

This had indeed been the case as Ms X's mother had a mastectomy when Ms X was a child and had recently died from a cancer on her ovary.

Ms X had the operation to remove the lump, and was informed that it had been 100 per cent successful, that no other treatment was required, and that there was nothing more to worry about. Ms X was reassured by this and felt quite well. However, within two years the lump returned. Again it was benign but, this time, a full mastectomy was needed. Once again she was told that the operation had been 100 per cent successful, no other treatment was required, and there was nothing more to worry about. This time, however Ms X did not find that statement so reassuring. Ms X was offered and accepted hypnosis to see if it might help to discover why she had developed a cancer at such a young age.

The technique described above was used to enhance Ms X's memory and feelings of early childhood experiences. Initially, two things were very clear: that she had been particularly close to her mother and that she was still very much grieving her mother's death. Over several weeks of hypnotherapy she continued to explore her early experiences, the effects they had on her, the decisions she had made in response to those events and how those decisions were still affecting her on a subconscious level, especially in relation to self-esteem, confidence and anxiety. During this time she had also been having bereavement counselling separately, until she was able to accept her mother's death and say a symbolic goodbye to her.

Results of hypnotic regression
By now Ms X was emotionally a much stronger and calmer person, with much improved self-esteem and confidence. When in hypnosis, she recalled the time her mother had a mastectomy. At the time

Ms X was seven years old and had been missing her mother because, unfortunately, she had been placed with an unsympathetic childminder, which made her situation even worse. To add to this, children were not allowed on the ward, so she could see her mother only through the window in the door.

Despite her young age, she was aware of the seriousness of her mother's illness and thought to herself that if anything were to happen to her mother she could not live without her, and so she too must die. Owing to the powerful emotions that went with this thought, the idea was engraved on her subconscious mind. Fortunately, her mother survived and lived until Ms X was 23. However, because of the immense grief Ms X felt when her mother died, that early belief that she too would die was activated, and so she developed the very same illness her mother had, at that time.

Outcome

The recall of this trauma meant that Ms X, while in hypnosis, could re-evaluate that early belief and, in effect, her subconscious that at 22 years old she could indeed live without her mother, and that the idea that she could not was to be removed. Interestingly, many of Ms X's anxiety symptoms were similar to the symptoms of her mother's illness: coughing, tiredness and so on. These all disappeared after she had been able to say goodbye to her mother.

At the time of writing, eight years has passed, and there has not been any recurrence of the cancer.

Discussion

At this point, reconsider the consultant's comment: "We do not know what causes it. We know it is not genetic, but it seems to run in families." (Recent work suggests that this is no longer thought to be so.) We suggest that it might be learned (copied) behaviour. Much human behaviour is gained from imitation. For example, one learns to walk and talk, mainly by observing our parents; and many of ones mannerisms are similarly learned, but without conscious effort. All this, and very much more, is achieved in early childhood. Is it so unlikely, then, that while we are busily absorbing all this wonderful material, the mind is also absorbing some negative processes, such as how ones parents behave in stressful and difficult situations, and how they cope when they become ill?

Consider again the thought of the young child: if anything were to happen to her mother she could not live without her. This raises another question: if a person wishes to die, is it possible that the subconscious mind can fulfil this wish? We have seen many examples in this book of the mind's positive effect in curing cancer, so we cannot be surprised to find it capable of a negative effect also if the wish is strong enough. Most people know of an old person who died shortly after the death of his or her partner. People say they died of a broken heart, or they lost the will to live.

Maxwell Maltz MD, in his book *Psycho-Cybernetics*,[2] describes a case study that illustrates how a simple idea can have a powerful negative effect on the body. Maltz had performed a minor cosmetic operation on Mr Russell's lower lip. Subsequently, in a heated argument, Mr Russell's partner announced that she was placing a "voodoo curse" upon him. This patient and his partner were born in the West Indies, where voodoo was practised, and as he noticed a small lump in his mouth he believed it to be the feared "African bug". Maltz describes how this man appeared to age twenty years in a few weeks.

On examination of the lump in Mr Russell's mouth, Maltz realised that it was a small piece of scar tissue from the operation that he had performed, which he then removed and showed to him. He noticed an immediate change in his posture and expression and the ageing process very quickly reversed.

"If you could have seen Mr Russell as I did, both before and after, you would never again entertain any doubts about the power of belief, or that an idea accepted as true from any source, can be every bit as powerful as hypnosis."

Case study 2
"I have never had so much wonderful attention in all my life" – Ms B, a cancer patient.

History of presenting symptoms

Ms B was in her early thirties. She had a history of an active cancer involving her breast, and surgery with apparent remission. Further cancer of the breast and surgery followed, with apparent remission. Later, tumours came to her back, shoulders and hip and her general condition was deteriorating. Ms B had had an unhappy life working as a civil servant in the UK's Department of Social Security. Her partial deafness had given her a loud voice with which she alienated herself from study and social groups. Ms B was plain-looking and clumsy, physically and socially. She had had a series of boyfriends but there were also periods without. Many were themselves disadvantaged socially. When she was invited to participate in our work with cancer sufferers she was single.

Results of hypnotic regression

Our first session consisted of general introductions and Ms B told of her cancer. In counselling, she was very general and vague, so we moved on to the hypnosis for which a quite long progressive relaxation was used. Towards the end, some twenty minutes later, I said, "You are becoming stronger every day." At this she jumped and came out of hypnosis. Some superficial conversation followed and Ms B left.

I puzzled over her reaction to my statement and concluded that the idea of getting stronger was in some way not comfortable to her.

A week later we had our second session. Again, in counselling she was quite general and vague, mostly talking about her week. In hypnosis I noticed that she seemed to resist letting herself relax. She kept fighting, making excuses to move and talk about inconsequential matters. Again, towards the end of the session I said, "You are becoming stronger every day." This time she made a more subtle jerk, but still her level of relaxation was reduced.

These two sessions implied to us that we should offer counselling alone, because of the obvious resistance to hypnotic regression and the suggestion that she would become strong. During the following two sessions of counselling, she put emphasis on the loneliness of her life and her forlorn expectation that she would fail to find an attractive man for a partner. Life seemed to have nothing to offer to Ms B.

The next session included a more direct question as to whether Ms B would really like to get better. Although reluctant to respond, she said that she feared that this would mean she had to give up the attention she was receiving as a consequence of her illness. "I have never had so much wonderful attention in all my life," she added. Two more sessions followed in which alternative ways of gaining attention, without the threat of death, were explored. Death was mentioned on several occasions, and once she was bluntly told by the therapist, "You will receive little attention when you are six feet under." This did not result in distress, but the equally blunt assertion that life had little to offer her.

Outcome

It would seem that Ms B had accepted that the attention she received as a cancer patient was wonderful, even if this meant an early death. Ms B finally began to cancel appointments, and then, later, she said she was too unwell to come any more. She was finally hospitalised. We visited her in hospital and found her welcoming, thankful and cheerful, with an implied expectation of further useful treatment. She died some weeks later.

Discussion

This case is a clear example of what Freud would call the death wish. Ms B rejected the idea of hypnosis to explore subconscious conflicts, find reasons for her cancerous growth or to receive suggestions for healing. We were never given the opportunity to explore Ms B's childhood and perhaps find reasons for the socially unacceptable characteristics that led to her loneliness. We expected a subconscious death wish, not one so conscious and accessible.

Because of this experience, we are alerted to cries, however disguised or muted, for attention. We both cringe now at the dismissal by parents and teachers of what they call attention seeking. The phrase "Ignore them – they're only seeking attention" comes from those who do not understand the importance of the need such behavioural signals.

We think all people need lots of loving attention – when they are young, especially. It is considered a sin to seek attention in some parts of our culture. We think that, psychologically, attention is essential to our health. We emphatically reject the idea that a child can be spoiled with attention. Life's experience will show the child that they cannot have what they want all the time without parents having to teach them this by deliberate withdrawal.

Case study 3
"I was a horrible child" – Ms F a cancer patient.

History of presenting symptoms
A woman of about 36 years (Ms F) came to us about marital diffi-culties. The main problem, as presented, was financial. Shortly after counselling began, Ms F reported that she had thyroid trou-ble. She showed a scar on her throat and spoke of radium treat-ment. It appeared to us that Ms F was someone who could benefit from hypnotherapy. The treatment consisted of weekly sessions of approximately two and a half hours, comprising one hour of client-centred counselling followed by an hour and a half of hypnotic regression therapy, for four months in the first instance.

Results of hypnotic regression
Ms F was very open and responsive from the beginning. Memories of past events and traumas were enhanced and reviewed while she was in hypnosis. She had an immense store of memories and imag-inative dreams to draw upon while in hypnosis, and a profusion of enhanced visualisations. The visualisations were self-directed and often related to her life experience, and were interpreted by Ms F. Other factors include the following:

1. As a child, Ms F hated her mother's new partner.

2. In hypnosis she explained that she became an asthmatic by copying it from a girl she knew, for attention. She did not get the attention, but the asthma stayed. This memory came as a great shock as it was something she had completely forgot-ten. The imitation had become a reality. Once she realised she

had caused the asthma herself, she also realised she could dispense with it. She has been clear of it ever since.

3. She was preoccupied with her partner's "meanness", which was a focus for the unsatisfactory nature of their relationship.

4. Her resistance to getting well was demonstrated during the first session when, on the point of coming out of hypnosis, the suggestion was made, "You will be stronger every day, fit and well." Ms F shot up and out of hypnosis.

Ms F early on stated in hypnosis, "I was a horrible child." It was obvious that she suffered from low self-esteem and self-hatred, and had a habit of putting herself down. She would do this latter action, Ms F said "to get there first, before anyone else can criticise me". These were the things that emerged, quite quickly, in hypnosis. Not wishing to upset others, she became submissive, pretending that insults did not hurt her. Her inability to express her feelings was soon overcome as the therapy progressed. She came to acknowledge that withholding her feelings was damaging to her. Repressed anger and upset were visualised in hypnosis as a World War Two mine. We were impressed by the power this image had in her imagination. For example, in one hypnotic session she said she was in the water with a mine – "a big round thing with spikes all over". She said the mine was inside her and there to keep things inside her. The mine Ms F reported seeing was as she saw it symbolic of something inside of her – the cancer. The mine did not like her swearing, made her hold her temper in and stopped her shouting and swearing. She explained that she could get the mine to go away in several ways. It could just drift away or disappear, or be taken away by a boat with a crane. However, she was reluctant to remove it, saying that she could make it come and go. The mine was her cancer. She kept saying that she was not afraid of the mine. She also said that others had noted on the remarkable lack of fear that she had of her cancer. Ms F eventually acknowledged that the mine was not effective enough, and that there were better ways of dealing with her suppressed anger. Eventually, the mine was defused.

In hypnotic regression Ms F recalled that, at the age of about eleven, she arrived home from six weeks in Austria, on the day her father died. Although her father was not very nice to her, he was an important figure in her life and affections. She did not have the opportunity to say goodbye to him then, nor had she since, and therefore, for over twenty years, she had been suffering from an unresolved state of grief. While in hypnosis she took the opportunity to say goodbye to her father and felt very relieved.

Another trauma that she addressed occurred when she was sixteen. It centred on a kidnapping, of her and a friend by a group of male peers. Ms F managed to escape, but bravely returned to rescue her friend. She said this was the first time she had told anyone of the incident. Keeping secrets is a strain for most of us. Guilt about such secrets can erode our spirit. Sharing it with a person who will be empathic and nonjudgmental can give immediate, and often permanent, relief. This can enable one to move on, forgive oneself and finally resolve such burdens.

We propose that Ms F's cancer seemed to have been caused by suppressed upset and anger, and an inability to express these feelings, which started in early childhood and continued through adolescence to marriage and motherhood. She had always been an over-anxious person with a desire not to upset others. This established a life-long habit of emotional repression, which she eventually turned upon herself.

In her present adult life, a major source of stress was her relationship with her partner, and the question of whether she should leave him. Many weeks of therapy continued with self-esteem enhancement and the release of resentments and anger. At times there seemed to be great improvements in her relationship with her partner, but then the arguments would start again. Ms F came to recognise that she did not communicate with her partner in a positive way, and she seemed unable to break this habit for a long time. For example, she was unable to recall the last time she had said something pleasant to her partner although he had paid her compliments. Ms F had been angry at the suggestion of a former counsellor that her partner was the victim, because she would not allow him to go to hospital with her or to attend therapy on Fridays with her. She became quite indignant on the Friday subject – "*It was my business,*" said Ms F. Perhaps her freedom and independence day?

Our discussion led to a comparison between her partner's financial meanness and her emotional meanness. As the weeks went by, one other significant event occurred, within the context of whether she should stay with her partner or not. Ms F was asked, while in hypnosis, what would make her happy. She replied that she already had it: Her children and her home.

In hypnosis, Ms F had some quite amazing, imaginative journeys – self-directed – from New York to Australia, past the Statue of Liberty, walking on the bottom of the Atlantic through the *Titanic*. This imagery was linked to her grandfather, who had been a sailor and had died at sea. She was still grieving for him, and through this imagery was able to say goodbye.

In one session, another hypnotic visualisation took us to the Sidney Opera House, and to *Star Trek* and the USS *Enterprise*, with Captains Kirk and Picard arguing about the captain's chair. She told them off "nicely, of course" and sat in the captain's chair. Then, because they did not have enough power, she left the set to talk to the story writers and tell them off "not nastily, of course". We see in this her attempt to assert herself and to take control of her life, with echoes of the past – her not wishing to upset anyone.

We made a hypnotic tape designed for Ms F's daily use. When we asked her, many weeks later, she admitted that she had listened to it only once. She said that it was difficult for her to find the time. She seemed to have little sense of responsibility for her own health, and a lack of motivation to become well. Months later we were still trying to get her to use the tape, but she was rarely making the effort. Despite this, Ms F's health improved and her self-development progressed with the continuing hypnotherapy.

Outcome
A dramatic increase in assertiveness was noted, as her attitude towards her partner changed. She became less subservient, less dependent and then more independent in herself.

There was also a change in her clothes colour, from black to white and beige. We saw this as a sign of some freeing of her spirit from depression. An increase in self-esteem was demonstrated by less negativity and more optimism towards herself and her future; and greater enthusiasm for the therapy as it proceeded.

Later in the therapy, Ms F had new imagery. She was a winner in a series of game shows. In each show, a bit of herself was won until she won herself as a prize. She said she felt better about winning herself than if she had won a big prize – a car or similar item.

At another stage in therapy, Ms F said she felt stretched and twisted by a big stone sitting on top of a cream cake or walnut whirl, which was her. She went on to tell of more assertiveness and wanting flowers, but having no time to plant. She put a lot of emphasis on the fact that her partner was not going to change – she repeated this several times. She wanted to be more positive about the future.

She mentioned that we called her Fiona and that she was used to being called by either of two nicknames, which she preferred when she did not like herself. Now she likes to hear the full version, and says, "I like myself now."

Discussion

Suggestions made under hypnosis were:

- assertive
- stress-free
- immune system full strength
- diet more healthy – less chocolate

As we write this, Ms F is having quarterly checks at the hospital and seems to be re-establishing a good relationship with her partner. No further therapeutic meetings are scheduled. Her self-esteem has significantly improved, but still does not show a lively will for good health. The sitting-on-the-fence aspect of her relationship is a sign that more therapy is needed.

Ms F's creative and virile imagination has given us one of the most dramatic and widespread journeys that we have experienced in a hypnotic client. It has been for us an illustration of how a self-directed exploration can produce the richest symbolism: Pointers to the trauma we have experienced, and images we can use to help us explain and resolve the hurt. It also illustrates for us how children's emotional, physical affection, (cuddles, touching and stroking) and intellectual needs (valuing and listening on the one hand, with the child's point of view in mind and, on the other hand, sensitive explanations of separation, death and loss) may not be understood even by caring adults. How do we make time for these things in the busy life of a modern parent?

Case study 4
"Although no one died! Can grief cause cancer?"

This is a case study of BM as client and DF as therapist.

History of presenting symptoms
Mr B, a sixty-plus male, during a week in March 1995, of hard physical work installing a fire and a washing machine, a subfloor and a wall of shelves, and a variety of smaller jobs, began to experience stomach pains. These pains would be relieved, so he could continue work, by exercises designed to disperse abdominal congestion. As the week progressed he realised that his bowel stopped working, most unusual, as daily movement was his norm.

During his journey home from Scotland, in the train his discomfort increased and he visited his doctor the next day. After his examination, the doctor said he would send him to hospital, but that he would probably be sent home because he would not be classed as an emergency. The client had a full-time job and had not had more than five or ten days away from work in the previous forty years. The last visit to his doctor was seven years previously. Next day, back at home, he was obviously weaker and the doctor visited him and immediately sent for the ambulance. That evening he had a piece of his bowel removed with a golf-ball-sized obstruction that was found to be cancerous. Recovery was uneventful and his life resumed as before within two or three months.

Results of hypnotic regression
Therapy commenced while he was in hospital when he recounted a dream to his therapist. The client was on his way to work involving

a walk through the environs of his establishment. The ground was fissured with cracks all over the place, not dangerous in size, but continuously bridged in the cracks by lightning flashes. He was not frightened by them but very puzzled. He kept asking passers-by what they meant, but to no enlightenment. They were blasé about this phenomenon and the client insisted that he should take time out to investigate it. There seemed to be a link between the dream and the cause of the cancer. We interpreted the lightning flashes as the cancer and the puzzle represented the uncertainty as to the cause of the tumour.

Therapy started in the client's home. There was no obvious reason for the illness. During hypnotic regression therapy it soon became apparent that an ideal employment opportunity had been lost. His boss had eliminated his department, but not his job and the loss of job satisfaction had grieved the client deeply. This had happened twice. An alternative employment with a new college pursuing the work that he had had with his previous job was also terminated. This grief was exacerbated because the client blamed himself for not being able to prevent the loss. He was further damaged by a sense of political impotence and fury at the government of the time for what he considered hypocrisy.

Hypnotic therapy brought these events to centre stage. Mr B realised that the effects of the grief, anger and depression on his immune system was almost certainly the cause of his cancer. Although no one had died, bereavement counselling was appropriate, as the losses felt were profound and disabling.

Outcome
Weekly hypnotic counselling was continued for five or six months, supplemented by the daily use of a personal hypnotic healing tape from the therapist. The client worked through the recognised grieving process. Six years and three clear colonoscopies, showed that all was well.

Discussion
What healed him? Therapy? His immune system? Was it the operation? A combination of all three? What we do claim is that the

therapy removed the burden of grief from his immune system. This indicates an emotional/psychological cause behind the symptom of cancer.

A revised formula

Reading through these case studies gave us food for thought, and we looked for common elements. They seem to be unresolved grief for loss of a parent, or career, and deprivation of an affectionate childhood or love in an adult life. Low self-esteem, illustrated by self-hatred and self-blame, so often a recurring theme, is the focus of so many of our therapeutic exercises.

We thought that perhaps a formula could be offered to fit these cases of illness (as Gindes offers to us for the creation of the hypnotic state) as follows:

Lack of love and attention in childhood
(love not demonstrated verbally, emotionally or physically)

+

Unresolved bereavement or
loss in childhood or later

+

Low self-esteem

+

Self-blame

=

Illness, through an immune system weakened
by the loss of will to live.

Chapter 6

Therapeutic Hypnosis – Other Uses

Conditions Treated by Hypnosis

In 1906, Dr Auguste Forel[1] was able to compile a long list of conditions that had been found to respond to hypnotic suggestion. It included pains of all descriptions (especially headache, neuralgia, sciatica and toothache), sleeplessness, functional and organic paralysis, chlorosis (anaemia), menstrual problems, loss of appetite, all nervous digestive disturbances, constipation, some kinds of diarrhoea, dyspepsia, alcoholism, drug addiction, rheumatism, lumbago, stammering, seasickness, bedwetting, chorea (nervous twitching of the body) anxiety disorders, phobias and "bad habits of all kinds".

This list has stood the test of time, and today hypnosis is commonly used to treat all of these conditions. Currently, we could expand the list even further to include asthma, eczema, depression, sexual problems, ME, stammering, smoking, weight reduction, anorexia, bulimia and shyness. In fact, we would go so far as to say that most medical conditions could be treated with hypnosis, and many medical treatments enhanced with hypnosis. The list is so long that we fear it looks like an advert for patent medicine! However, if one considers the success in terminal cancer cases, it is not surprising that its effectiveness is demonstrated in so many other fields.

The most astonishing thing about hypnosis is that it continues to achieve significant success, even when traditional medicine has had limited results. We mentioned haemophilia, for instance, in Chapter 2. Other examples that we have witnessed, or assisted with, concern childbirth, pregnancy (morning sickness, dietary obsessions, heat discomfort, tiredness) and breast enlargement (without surgery or implants). These have been helped with a simple hypnotic procedure that has proved highly successful. In the case of childbirth, as well as producing a highly efficient natural anaesthetic that does not affect the baby, hypnosis can also reduce the delivery time. One gynaecologist who regularly uses hypnosis for this purpose told us that her average delivery time is two hours.[2]

The treatment of burns is another area where hypnosis has been very successful, even with third-degree burns. A simple procedure can be employed in which the patient is hypnotised as soon as possible after the accident, when it is suggested that the patient feel cool and comfortable. Not only is there a reduction in pain but, astonishingly, there is no swelling to the burned area. This means that the healing process is much quicker and scarring is also significantly reduced. One of us, DF, remembers treating a man with cerebral palsy. He was hypnotised once a week for about a year. By the end of this time, he had greater control of his body movements and his speech had improved by between 60 and 70 per cent.[3]

Practical Psychology

One area in which hypnosis has proved to be most valuable is that of practical psychology. Its effectiveness in reducing stress and increasing confidence and self-esteem, can produce profound changes in a person's day-to-day existence, enabling them to overcome shyness, attract a partner, perform well in work and at job interviews, and so on.

Such personal improvement can be extended to the development of natural talent. Sports people and musicians often use hypnotism for this purpose. Recognising the potential of hypnosis to enhance everyday life, we have found it worthwhile to provide weekend courses in self-hypnosis, two or three times a year, for the past five or six years. A former student remarked to us that she still used the technique, and had found it very helpful in relieving the symptoms of hay fever. Such comments are very gratifying. Another of our students recently ran up and flung her arms around one of us, exclaiming, "I have found my serenity." We have lost count of the number of times people have told us that their lives have been dramatically changed by our courses.

Two short case studies:

1. A person, whose self-confidence was low for many years, had not been able to obtain a job appropriate to her abilities. After a self-hypnosis course, her confidence increased. Later, she informed us that she had completed a successful interview for a prestigious job.

2. One woman, who came on the course out of general interest, later reported to us her success in reducing eczema, overcoming her fear of heights and having a comfortable childbirth. She concluded that the course had changed her life.

Although the course is easy, and suitable for people of all ages, it should be stressed that not all conditions are amenable to self-hypnosis and may require facilitation by a trained therapist, particularly if the cause of the problem is unclear or arises from a traumatic experience.

Childbirth

Childbirth is an area where hypnosis could be used most beneficially. Hypnosis (and self-hypnosis training) could be offered to every pregnant woman. The cost of this would be insignificant when compared with that of current medical procedures. Childbirth is a very painful experience for many women, possibly needlessly so.[4]

Case study

A woman in her mid-twenties (Ms P) wanted to have her first baby naturally at home. She had previously attended a self-hypnosis course and asked one of us if we would facilitate her with hypnosis. As is often the case, Ms P had heard many horror stories of the pain of labour, stitches and all the things that can go wrong. Listening to these episodes had made her anxious and frightened of the supposed ordeal. Therefore, in the first instance, hypnosis was used to relieve her fear and to promote confidence in her body's natural ability to give birth. She soon became more calm and relaxed.

It is unwise to give direct hypnotic suggestion for the removal of pain, as this may deprive us of a good warning sign should something go wrong. In the treatment of Mrs P, therefore, suggestions were made only for "safe, natural, smooth, comfortable and easy birth ". As she had previously attended a self-hypnosis, course she was given a hypnotic audiotape with these suggestions for her daily use (we do not recommend any hypnotic tape for people with no knowledge of hypnosis).

All mothers have an ability to communicate with their unborn baby (Dr Thomas Verny, the author of a book called *The Secret Life of the Unborn Child*,[5] calls this sympathetic communication) and we decided to try hypnosis as a means of enhancing this communication. As this was an experimental procedure, we wanted to use as many safeguards as possible, so the first suggestion given was, "The following ideas will only take effect if they are good for you and your baby's health and wellbeing, at all levels of self, physically, emotionally, and spiritually. Good health for you, and your baby, at all levels is the main priority."

The following suggestions were then given. "In a way that is good, beneficial, and progressive for you and your baby at all levels of self, now, while you are in this state of relaxed hypnosis, you have the opportunity to enhance your ability to communicate with your baby. You can converse so easily and effectively with your baby. It's just as if there were a telephone line connected between you and your baby." DF then asked Ms P if she could do this. She nodded positively. There were a few minutes of quiet while she sent messages of reassurance and love to her baby. It was easy to see an increase in the baby's movements. She then said that she was feeling warm and cosy and that she was getting a feeling of belonging coming from her baby. She added that the baby felt happier and more secure. She then began to describe what the baby looked like. At the end of the hypnosis Ms P described her experience as wonderful. This procedure was used several times.

Ms P reported that the birth started early in the morning. Her spouse phoned the midwife while Ms P sat comfortably and awaited her arrival. The midwife came shortly afterwards. The baby arrived twelve hours later. Throughout the labour Ms P remained relaxed and comfortable and had no medical anaesthetic. The baby boy weighed about 3.6 kilos (8 pounds 1 ounce). Considering his size, she was delighted that she did not need any stitches. It was not until after the birth that the midwife mentioned that the baby had been in the posterior position (baby's back to mother's back). This usually makes for a more painful birth than normal, as the baby has to turn a half-circle before it can be delivered (the correct position for the baby is called the anterior position – baby's back to mother's stomach).

Approximately two and a half years later Ms P became pregnant again. She had been so pleased with the effect of hypnosis in the delivery of the first child that she requested hypnotic assistance once more. The procedure for the second birth was the same as the first. However, this time, in the third month of pregnancy, she was told that again the baby was in the posterior position and she wondered whether it would be possible to place the baby correctly. And, after careful consideration, we decided it was worth a try. Fortunately, Ms P had the same midwife, whose knowledge of hypnosis allowed her to discuss the idea with us without any unreasonable fear or prejudice. She told us that it was impossible but that she had no objection to our trying. Once again Ms P was hypnotised, using the same safety precautions as before, and communication was established with baby via the same imaginary telephone line. This time however, she *asked* the baby to turn into the anterior position, while, at the same time, she visualised its happening. Instantly the baby started making large movements.

On the midwife's next visit, with some surprise she confirmed that the baby had turned to the desired position, which was maintained until the start of labour. Unfortunately, during the 24-hour labour the baby turned a full 360-degree circle before delivery. Babies in the anterior position normally rotate only a one-third circle during labour. Afterwards the midwife deduced that the shape of Ms P's pelvis would accept a baby only in the posterior position. It is recommended, therefore, that anyone using hypnosis for this purpose check the shape of the pelvis first.

Although the labour was slow, Ms P was comfortable throughout the first stage, mostly chatting and watching television, needing no anaesthetic. By the second stage she had become tired and required gas and air. This time she delivered a baby boy weighing a whopping 4.4 kilos (9 pounds 12 ounces) and, again, needed no stitches.

It seems likely to us that, as hypnotic suggestion can turn a foetus from posterior to anterior position, it could also be used to turn a breech baby to a normal position.

Pain Relief

The history of hypnosis is full of accounts of major operations carried out using hypnotic suggestion for anaesthesia and comfort. Current medical literature has many examples of surgical and dental operations carried out without drugs or anaesthetics (see Chapter 1).

There are also many examples of hypnotic relief, for the serious side effects of drugs. In our self-hypnosis courses we discuss the value of pain as a warning sign when something is wrong. Therefore, if the pain comes from an unknown source, it should be examined before any attempt is made to remove it.

The BBC documentary *Hypnosis and Healing* shows a young girl having her cavities drilled out under hypnosis. The procedure was completed without any anaesthetic or any other form of pain control.

Stammering

The speech of a person with a stammer has the form of a crying child trying to get its words out, and generally, stammering begins when a child is very upset and trying to explain what has upset them and no one will listen. Sometimes the child is disciplined (often unfairly, although with good intentions). The shock to the child of this experience may stay with them, in the form of difficulty in getting words out. In adulthood the person has often forgotten the original experience. Hypnotic regression to the time of the trauma can allow the person to review the experience and to release repressed emotions. Once this has been done, and with a consequent increase in confidence, the stammer often disappears permanently.

One case involved a young man who had been a stammerer most of his life. Having attended a course specifically for stammerers in Scotland, which had helped him a lot, he came to one of us (BM) for therapy to complete the removal of his affliction. Conflict with a domineering boss had rekindled his stammer, but, in addition, he was coming to a very significant time in his life, and wanted a therapeutic atmosphere in which to air and review with a therapist his hesitant decisions.

The regression

In the first session, before he entered hypnosis, we discussed his childhood when he had been envious of his two older step-brothers, who had another father and home, and a much more privileged lifestyle. In hypnotic regression, he recalled his childhood and was visibly moved by his feelings of loss, anger and deprivation. Tears ran down his cheeks, and he did not seek to hide his feelings, or apologise for them. He said that he had not realised how much it had affected him. This seemed to be a significant piece of self-knowledge made conscious. After a while the therapist asked if he wished to explore further.

After a little while longer the therapist perceived the patient's weariness and asked him again. He said that he had explored enough for now. Before bringing him out of hypnosis, the therapist read out the following suggestions agreed beforehand: "I'm calmer now and in the presence of my supervisor. My confidence is growing and spreading to all parts of my life, and not only those areas where I am seen as strong and competent. My determination to solve my problems is growing. My life is increasingly full of my new confident self, with no room for jealousy. I express my feelings of anger, sadness, jealousy and envy, and a sense of deprivation, so as to free myself from their unwelcome effects. My self-esteem is growing every day. My calmness is growing every day." He was then brought out of hypnosis and the session came to a close.

The second session started with his stating that he had had a good week, and that he had felt great relief from the previous week's hypnotherapy. In the subsequent regression he went back to an occasion when he was very young and had entered his mother's bedroom while his mother's lover was lying on the bed watching television. He was ordered out of the room because he had not knocked. He was terrified, and felt humiliated (even at 27 he would never enter a closed room without knocking). He then went forward to a time when he was fourteen and felt humiliated by his mother. He now feels hatred for her and cannot imagine forgiving her. He wants to add learning to forgive to his list of suggestions

By the third and final session his stammer had gone.

He had only three sessions of regression and review under hypnosis. He was then enabled to finish with a relationship that, in essence, had come to an end already (with a considerable degree of acceptance on both sides), leave an uncongenial job and accept another job thousands of miles away, which had been a 'hobby waiting to become a profession'. His last session was a song of happiness. "I just had to tell you," he said. For him it was a declaration of freedom. His life was opening up.

Conclusion

It may not be immediately obvious how these sessions of hypnotic regression removed his stammer. The process was in stages. First, he was able to recall his early traumatic experiences, which had terrified and humiliated him, taking away his self-esteem and confidence, resulting in his stammer. Second, as an adult, he could understand that he no longer needed to hold these feelings within him. Therefore, he was able to release the suppressed emotions. Third, free from feelings of fear and humiliation, he became calmer, his self-esteem and confidence returned, and the stammer disappeared.

Asthma

One of us (BM) many years ago, while on a visit to a friend, had a chest infection that required a visit to the local hospital at 4 a.m. After the inhalation of oxygen and various drugs, he recovered. Subsequent minor asthma attacks were treated with an inhaler. This was long before his acquaintance with hypnosis, but he was forming a conviction that asthma could be treated with the mind alone.

He then decided that he would treat the next attack of tightness in the chest by lying down, clearing the mind of anxieties and planting the idea that relaxation would allow the chest to give up its tension. Eventually, he discarded the inhaler. Very occasionally the tightness returns and he recognises he needs to relax and slow down until the tension has gone. Looking back now we realise that this practice was self-hypnosis allowing the body and mind to heal.

ME or Chronic Fatigue Syndrome (Myalgic Encephalomyelitis)

ME is a crippling disability, sometimes thought to be a reaction to a virus infection, in which fatigue, muscular pains and exhaustion rule the person's life, preventing them from working and living a normal life. Great controversy on the subject still goes on. Some experts say it does not exist. Many sufferers just suffer. We believe the disease is a response to a subconscious need for rest from the trials of life. Life has become too burdensome. Pleasure and satisfaction have gone. The subconscious mind demands a rest, but society and the conscious mind demand continuation of 'normality' and the affairs of life. In this sort of conflict the subconscious mind is bound to win, making the subject truly ill, forcing him/her to rest.

As therapists, we see the need to treat this condition very seriously. We would expect to find conflict between the needs and expectations of the individual and those of society. Hypnosis provides a mechanism for communication with the subconscious mind enabling both therapist and client to determine the relevant factors.

Therapy provides an opportunity for the expression and validation of the subject's feelings. These feelings, in some cases long suppressed, need to be understood. In this way, a new lifestyle, that meets the needs of the subconscious mind, can be prepared. We would expect to see greater assertiveness and self-esteem, more time for relaxation and pleasure, and an increased general awareness of their individual needs. Once recognition of need has been established there is usually a continuous improvement. Symptoms are relieved, and the full life can be enjoyed. Society tends to neglect the real needs of the individual to enjoy and have satisfaction in life, which are seen as selfish, leading to feelings of guilt, exhaustion and illness.

Case Study

An attractive woman in her fifties agreed to hypnotherapy because of her depression and lack of motivation.

She had had a family of four children and an exacting job, and had separated from her husband to free herself from a rather repressive relationship. Her attempts to re-establish herself as a professional woman were hampered by depression and extreme fatigue. She had the symptoms of ME for 15 years before it was diagnosed. This was followed by a further four years of bad health, during which she set her aim at facing her demons, one by one. She undertook 32 weekly 90 minute sessions of group therapy in the Psychology Department of a Psychiatric Hospital. She gained strength and confidence from the support of those in her team. She found the skilful facilitation, throughout the programme, by a woman psychotherapist significant for her personal development, Some improvement was achieved, but the treatment was time limited.

She had hypnotherapy several times a month, with BM, for several months, which included positive affirmations and regression to free her from subconscious disabling loyalties, self-denigratory habits, and to sever the disabling influence of her ex-husband. She became positively motivated and divorced her husband, which she considered was a milestone in her bid for freedom.

She now holds a responsible position in commerce, and her own house and mortgage, and represents her firm in public in many situations. She gives active support to her children and grandchildren. She acknowledges that her present outlook owes elements to all the influences over the past years, and to her own openness to embrace different ways to grow. She has an ambitious, but realistic personal development programme.

Chapter 7

Emotional Health

In Chapter 3 we discussed how depression can cause adults and children to become physically and sometimes terminally ill. In this chapter we attempt to give further insight into the causes of depression, and present some ideas on how to avoid it.

Major emotional stress arises from the sum of a number of relatively insignificant factors that, building up over a period of time, become an unhealthy burden on the individual. Once a person has reached this level, even tiny problems seem huge. In an attempt to justify their problem, the client has a tendency to say, "I *should* have done this" or "I *should* have said that". We refer to this as "should disease". It is, in simple terms, a guilt trip. When a person starts to punish him/herself by these internal accusations, the immune system becomes exhausted, and he/she can become physically ill, from an apparently organic cause – a virus or bacterium – or from a carcinogenic substance. In many people we find that the effect of these guilt feelings can make them dislike themselves – indeed, it is possible that they may even reach a stage where they actually hate themselves.

The Effects of Bereavement

One major source of emotional stress is the loss of a loved one. Our society does not always allow us time to grieve. Generally, we are offered a day or two, or even a week, off work and then we are expected to get on with our lives as though nothing had happened. This is totally unrealistic. Bereavement is a very significant shock to the system. People who have not suffered such a loss find it difficult to understand the intensity of the emotion involved. Often, when someone close to us dies, we have a tendency to detach ourselves from our emotions and delay experiencing the full intensity of grief. Such self-protection is necessary, in order that we may carry on with the banal activities of day-to-day living. This state of

111

mind, a sort of psychological numbness, can continue for years, especially if there is a tendency to keep very busy.

In the period immediately after bereavement, friends, children, workmates will see us when we are numb and think we are fine, much to their relief. However, when this stage eventually passes, feelings of depression can emerge. If a long period of time has passed, this can be confusing and people sometimes do not realise that our depression is caused by unresolved grief. Often after the loss of a loved one there can be a tendency for a person to blame him/herself with thoughts like "If only I had not gone to work that day"; "I *should* have been there"; "I *should* have done more". In some cases people can punish themselves emotionally and may even suffer the same physical symptoms that their loved one suffered before death.

A further difficulty arises when the bereaved person experiences the paradox of anger and a sense of loss at the same time. Anger arises against the dead person for leaving them alone, which, not surprisingly, can also lead to guilt feelings. The "don't speak ill of the dead" taboo still operates. Relief comes when the grieving person is supported through their loss, and enabled to talk and cry about the loved one and, eventually, to say a symbolic goodbye. This is never easy. After all, no one wants to let go of someone special but until this happens the depression continues – and may get worse – until the bereaved person is almost forced, by the intensity of their depression, to take action. Once relief has been achieved, the depression can disappear overnight, like magic.

We generally recommend writing a goodbye letter to the departed, which can be taken to the resting place or put somewhere special. Many people have told us that, once they have done this, they feel, in some spiritual way, closer to the person. They also tell us that they can look at his/her picture again, and go to the resting place and talk to him/her, without crying or feeling depressed.

An Invisible Form of Child Abuse

At what age can a person start to dislike him- or herself? This can start in early childhood. Most adults are disgusted by physical and sexual child abuse. But there is another form of child abuse, which, because it is invisible (there are no scars to be a seen), and because its effects may persist throughout the whole of the victim's life, may be considered at least as serious. We are talking about emotional child abuse. It may be defined as anything that damages a child's self-esteem or self-image. For example: depriving them of cuddles, ignoring them, telling them not to cry or show emotions, encouraging them to feel guilty ("It's your fault"), calling children stupid or silly, telling them not to "tell tales" when they have been hurt. People then wonder why children commit suicide after being bullied. Even when bullies get the blame, the victims have sometimes been made so vulnerable by emotional abuse that they have been sensitised to the point of despair.

Generally, adults simply don't listen to children. Take the example of going to school. When a child says, "I don't want to go to school", the child will usually be pressured to go anyway. Why? First, there is a legal requirement; then, there is the working parent's need to go to work; but, overall, there is the assumption that it is in the child's best interests to go. One of us remembers an occasion when a child who did not want to go to school was allowed to stay home without any fuss. As the day wore on, the child, while chatting to the parent casually, without prompting began to tell of what amounted to bullying. Immediate action through the headmaster led to a resolution – and no further reluctance to go to school. If the child had been *made* to go that day, who knows what the outcome might have been?

The vast majority of colleges and universities employ counsellors, yet relatively few schools employ them on a permanent basis. Obviously, children don't get depressed. They are simply being naughty, seeking attention, have behaviour problems, or are withdrawn!

In Britain, in particular, we have a tendency to set impossible goals for children, especially when we are in public. "Don't make a noise"; "Don't get dirty"; "Sit still"; "Be good"; "Don't embarrass me". All these, we must have heard. Yet the child never manages to be good enough. One of us once heard a young girl in a supermarket crying, "Mummy, I want to be good." People expect children to act like adults.

One of us recently read the school report of a child aged four, who was described as "immature" by his teacher. He was obviously late handing in his PhD thesis! All this simply says to children, "We don't care (about you). Just be quiet." Is it, then, a wonder that there is so much anger and violence in our schools? And what is to be done about it? The traditionalists say, "we need more discipline and curfews." "Oh yes!" chorus the more tolerant, because they have no alternative. "Oh no!" say those with more faith in their children, who, when they behave in what others would call a naughty way, react differently. Such people do not pretend they like the behaviour, but they do not treat the child as unpleasant, repulsive, a nuisance or worse.

We have seen children of one or two years old, being hit hard because they were tired, hungry, bored or ignored. If we try to listen more carefully, to verbal and body languages, we are likely to get a better understanding of the situation, and then react more positively to the child's message, with respect and tender loving care. We can share with them our own feelings about a situation by saying, "I feel upset" or "I'm getting angry now". Some years ago, one of us (DF), in a counselling class discussing parenting of young children, was asked how he disciplined his child of two years old, when his behaviour was upsetting. His reply was, "I do nothing, but tell him I'm upset, and hope he cares enough about my feelings to stop." The class laughed, saying that this would never work. But one woman agreed to try it with her six-year-old. Initially, she came back saying, with some amazement, that it had been very effective. A few weeks later she complained that it had now failed, because the child was telling her that she, the child, was getting upset. David said, "Good, that was the point of the exercise."

Encouraging children to express their feelings helps develop a mutual respect between them and their parents. If we want children or, indeed, anyone else to respect our feelings, we must also respect theirs. To emphasise the value of this newly learned skill, David asked the class to practise counselling their children, without asking any questions. This resulted in one woman saying, of her nine-year-old, "It's opened a can of worms. He's unhappy and being bullied at school. I learned more about him than I imagined was possible."

We believe that the vast majority of parents do the best they can, based on the knowledge and experience they have at the time, so we must emphasise that it is not our intention to accuse or blame anyone. After all, where do we learn to be parents? What does it say about a society that teaches its children a vast amount of facts that most forget as soon as they have finished their exams, yet totally ignores the most important lessons of all: making relationships work, being an effective parent and valuing of both others and ourselves.

Virginia Axline, in her book *Dibs in Search of Self*,[1] explains the case history of five-year-old Dibs. At the beginning of the book, Dibs did not talk and never left his chair. After some weeks, he crawled about a bit, but when anyone approached he would huddle up in a ball. He never looked into anyone's eyes and never answered when spoken to. His school attendance was perfect but he never took his own coat off and spent his time crawling, hiding under a table or behind the piano, and looking at books. Sometimes he seemed mentally retarded; sometimes he seemed superintelligent. Often he had temper tantrums. Every day, when his teacher, Hedda, came close, Dibs attacked her, striking, scratching, biting and screaming, "No go home." Sometimes another teacher, Jane, sat and read aloud and, although Dibs gave no obvious sign, she thought he listened. After two years in this private school, Dibs had made only minimal progress.

Teachers were baffled. A psychologist tried to test him several times, but eventually gave up. A paediatrician, after several attempts at assessment, threw up his hands in despair. "He's a strange one," he said. "Who knows? Mentally retarded? Psychotic? Brain-damaged? Who can get close enough to find out?" This exclusive school, on the Upper East Side of New York, took children from three to seven. Dibs's mother, having influence with the trustees, had obtained admission for her son. Dibs's father, a well-known scientist, had been seen by no one at the school.

In desperation, because they were unable to cope, the school asked Virginia Axline, a clinical psychologist, to give her opinion before they dismissed Dibs. The mother agreed to her seeing him. She said that she and her husband had accepted the fact that Dibs was probably mentally retarded or brain-damaged. Dibs's mother said that, if the school could no longer keep Dibs, she would like to be given the address of a private boarding school for mentally defective children.

Teacher Hedda exploded when hearing this, as she had sympathy for the child, as did teacher Jane. There was obviously something about Dibs that captivated their interests and feelings, despite the story of failure. They seemed to respect the child. Hedda went on to say, "His mother would rather believe he is mentally retarded than admit that he may be emotionally disturbed; and maybe she is responsible for it."

Axline observed Dibs at school. Axline's first impression of Dibs was that of a little boy crouched in a corner, head down, arms folded. When he selected a book and started reading a teacher went up to him and said, "Oh! I see you are looking at the bird book. Do you want to tell me about it, Dibs?" Dibs threw the book away and threw himself down on the floor. He lay face down, rigid and immobile. "I'm sorry," the teacher said, "I didn't mean to bother you, Dibs." She then approached Axline and said, "That was typical, we have learned not to bother him, but I wanted you to see." With difficulty, Axline arranged for Dibs to come for one hour a week of play therapy at the child guidance centre where she was conducting research.

The book is the story of the development of Dibs's relationship with Virginia Axline. On the first visit, Axline asked Dibs if he would go with her to the playroom at the end of the corridor, and he agreed. Dibs took her hand and spent the hour there with her. Axline said to Dibs, "You can see the toys and materials we have. You decide what you would like to do." Axline recounts that Dibs circled the room, that his step was heavy, and that there seemed to be no laughter or happiness in the child. Life for him was a grim business.

Dibs took items from the doll's house and spoke out their names. Axline responded. If he said, "This is a bed," Axline said, "This is a bed," or something similar, and acknowledged in this way anything he said and felt. Dibs began naming objects in the room. When he picked up the father doll and said "Papa," Axline replied, "It could be Papa." Dibs sat in silence. As Dibs played for an hour each week, his real self started to emerge. Axline let him do what he wanted and simply acknowledged what he was doing, making no judgments good or bad. On one occasion Dibs played with water in the sink. He placed his fingers over the tap and a fountain of water sprayed out into the room. "I, Dibs, can make the water a fountain and I can turn the colour of water blue." (Earlier, Dibs had washed out some blue ink.) "I can see you can," said Axline. He played with the water, turning it on with such force that it splashed out into the room again. "Oh boy! What fun!" said Dibs. "You're having lots of fun," said Axline. On another occasion Dibs set out plates, cups and saucers and a teapot and began a tea party. Dibs then, refilling the water pitcher, poured the water on the draining board, on the floor and on the table. Dibs said, "One great big sloppy splash all over the place." But he enjoyed every drop of it and every minute of it.

Dibs then returned to his play of pouring tea into seven cups, using a changed voice. He imitated perfectly the precise inflection and expression of his mother's voice. A tea-pouring procedure followed, with an authoritative comment on how it should be poured and arranged. He reached for the toast and upset one of the cups. He sprang up, a frightened expression on his face. "No more party," he said, and put all the cups on the shelf. "Stupid! Stupid! Stupid!" There were tears in his eyes. His voice choked. He expressed sorrow and acknowledged his negligence, but said, "I should have been more careful, but I am not stupid." Axline said, "You were careless, perhaps, but not stupid." "That's right," said Dibs, now with a smile. Dibs had successfully weathered this storm. The rest of the book is of a little boy, finding pleasure in his one hour a week of play therapy with a person-centred therapist, and becoming a happy child.

The therapist made no judgments, just acknowledged the validity of a little boy's feelings long enough for Dibs to accept them himself.

He was an imaginative, highly knowledgeable, very intelligent child, thought by his parents to be mentally defective and beyond their control. Virginia Axline responded to Dibs in a nondirective way, except to encourage him here and there in some co-operative behaviour, such as having him take off his own outdoor clothes when he arrived and put them on at the end of the session. By the time he was six he was re-integrated into his school. One wonders what would have happened to Dibs if he had not met Axline.

Where did Dibs's unhappy parents go wrong? They seemed unable to perceive his feelings, or perhaps they denied their validity. They expected a degree of precision from a child that would have been demanding from an adult. Fun and laughter seemed alien to their philosophy. Their discipline was harsh and proved humiliating for Dibs. Instead of improving him, it made him aggressive, withdrawn, caused him to act in a way that they saw as stupid, living up to their expectations. Such child abuse is not recognised, but it is, sadly, only too common. Many parents who do this would be horrified to see physical forms of abuse. They may be well meaning, but they lack parenting skills, through a lack of education. Alice Miller details much work on this subject in a series of books. One of her books is called the *Untouched Key*.[2]

The play sessions were used by Dibs to explore a range of issues, and Virginia Axline used the person-centred approach to counselling. This way is characterised by the three elements of unconditional positive regard, empathy and congruence: as developed by Rogers.[3]

Unconditional positive regard
Axline accepted Dibs as a worthwhile person, despite his behaviour. She was not judgmental. Unconditional positive regard means no punishment, but prizing of the individual, whatever their behaviour.

Empathy
Axline listened to Dibs and sought to understand the feelings behind his words, and then to communicate to Dibs her understanding of his feelings.

Congruence

Axline was honest, direct, warm and unpretentious, not hiding behind the "expert" cloak. What Axline thought and felt was evident in her expression to Dibs.

Once, during a counselling class discussing the water episode, the students became annoyed, thinking the therapist was at fault for not reprimanding the little boy. They seemed unable to perceive how the tightly controlled world that Dibs had endured for his few years of life had burdened him hugely; and how the freedom the therapist gave him for one hour per week validated his feelings and released him from his social prison.

We all internalise a set of values, which some call morals, but these are very different from person to person. We so easily condemn others who have different values from our own. Before you judge a child as good or bad, try this exercise:

1. First, list the ten most important values you live your life by.

2. Second, close your eyes and imagine you are six years old and make another list from a child's perspective. Once you have finished, look at the two lists and compare the differences.

3. Third, now ask yourself this question. Is a child good or bad, or does he/she simply have a different set of values?

How do we enhance a child's self-esteem?

We believe that much counselling does not uncover hidden stress, which are part of the burden cancer patients need to lose before their immune system can tackle the cancer. The following examples demonstrate how the Person-Centred approach to the non-directive exchanges can be successful in what appears to be intractable cases. When the hypnotherapy is Person-Centred, this appears to enhance its effectiveness.

This is not an easy thing to achieve, particularly as our own self-esteem may be, at best, a fragile flower. However, here are a few ideas.

First, take time to consider your own childhood. This often brings back painful memories you have tried hard to forget. If that is the case, discuss them with a counsellor. How did you feel when you were punished, ignored, or not given any attention? How were you comforted when you were upset? How did your parents show you they cared? How would you have liked your parents to treat you? Imagine you are a child now? How would you like to be treated?

Second, be positive. When a child is behaving in an undesirable way, take a few moments to consider why they are behaving in that way. Has something upset them? Do they want attention? Generally, attention seeking is thought to be a bad thing. We have often heard people say, "Ignore him, he's only seeking attention." But we all need positive attention. It tells us that we matter and that we are cared for.

Often, David's first child, when he was two or three years old, would create a disturbance when his father was having a conversation. "I would stop speaking and play with him for ten minutes or so. He would then go off and play happily by himself for thirty or forty minutes. After this he would again become troublesome, and I would once more give him some attention. Some would say that I had allowed him to manipulate me, but I believe them to be wrong."

Attention is a legitimate need, especially for children, that needs to be gratified. It is always a good idea to tell the child what you yourself would like rather than what you *don't* want. If, for example, your child is touching or doing something that is inappropriate, instead of saying, "Don't, don't, don't", offer a distraction, "Play with this" or "Play in that area". Praise is very important, so praise even little things. (If your response is disbelief, try it for yourself.)

Third, be honest with your children. Tell them how you feel. Say, "I'm pleased you said [or did] that" or "I'm getting upset now" or

"I'm getting cross now". Encourage them to verbalise their feelings rather than use misbehaviour to indicate that they are upset. Teach them to respect the feelings of others. We emphasise here that it is important to say "I feel" and not "You made me feel". The latter tends to instil guilty feelings, which will kill self-esteem.

Fourth, babies and children need physical contact and cuddles – the more the better. You can let babies and young children sleep in bed with you, if you take sensible precautions. If you are strongly against having a child in your bed, ask yourself why. It may be that you are overprotective of your territory, or a bit jealous of the attention the child is receiving from your partner. You may remember a lot of discussion in the media on the subject of cot death. One television documentary implicated cot mattresses. This theory was soon discredited and, shortly after, they brought out a second programme mainly blaming smokers. In the second programme, they stated that it had been proved that children who sleep in the same bed as their parents have a much deeper sleep than those that do not. They also said that in India, where it is the norm for babies to sleep in the same bed as their parents, there has never been a cot death, even though the weather is hotter and many people smoke.

The book *Three in a Bed*, by Deborah Jackson,[4] sets out all the arguments for and against having a baby in the parents' bed. Included is an article by the French birth pioneer Michel Odent who, in 1977, travelled to China. Odent says:

> Nobody understood my question; the concept of sudden infant death, or cot death, was apparently unknown among professionals and lay people in such different places as Peking, Hsian, Loyang, Nanking, Shanghai and Canton. Furthermore, I learned that Chinese babies sleep with their mothers, even in the most Westernised families, such as the families of interpreters. Ever since then I have held the view that even if it happens during the day, cot death is a disease of babies who spend their nights in an atmosphere-of-loneliness; and that cot death is a disease of societies where the nuclear family has taken over.

This atmosphere-of-loneliness theory is supported by research from hospitals in Scarborough and Sutton Coldfield. Drs A N Stanton and J R Oakley[5] studied illness in children who subsequently died suddenly and inexplicably. They found that a

121

significant proportion of babies who died from sudden-infant-death syndrome had earlier been admitted for a long stay in hospital.

In the British television programme *Tomorrow's World*, in 1978, there is included a time-lapse film of adults sleeping with their baby. Each time the baby rolls towards the parents, the parents move away in their sleep. However, parents under the influence of alcohol or other drugs may not retain this sensitivity.

If you are interested in these ideas on parenting, and have not yet thrown this book out of the window, you might like to read the list of books shown under references for chapter seven, that prompted these ideas.[6]

Alice Miller's books are easy to read, but thought provoking with regard for children and parenting. Try one, for example: *Breaking Down the Wall of Silence – to join the waiting child.*[7]

Finally, check your own self-esteem. You need it yourself if you want to help your children find their own.

Here are two exercises:

1. Write down quickly three things you are good at. How was that? Easy? Many people find it difficult. If we have low self-esteem it can be hard to acknowledge good things about ourselves. Can you acknowledge compliments graciously without denial?

2. Make a list of all the things you do not like about yourself. Then make a second list of the things you do like about your-self. Hopefully, the list of likes is longer than the list of dis-likes. If you are British, we suspect not.

If you have found the above exercises difficult, or have more dis-likes than likes, it means that you need to learn to be kind to yourself. We have observed that people tend to be much harder on themselves than they would be on a friend. For example, if a friend made a mistake of some kind, the chance is you would say something to the effect of, "Never mind, everyone makes mistakes.

Forget it." If, however, you made a similar error yourself, you would probably get angry with yourself, call yourself stupid and be unforgiving. People seem to want to be perfect, and set impossible standards for themselves. They emotionally beat themselves up when they fail to reach these unobtainable standards. It is much better to give yourself the same sort of comfort and advice that you would give to your best friend.

Check to see if the items that you don't like about yourself are just normal human frailties. If they are, cross them off the list. Also check for terms such as "lazy" or "selfish". If you consider yourself to be lazy or selfish, it is very likely that you are not, but have been manipulated into thinking this way by someone who wants to control you or wants you to live by their value system. A person who is truly selfish would not recognise this trait in themselves.

If there is something that makes you angry with yourself, ask yourself if you would forgive it of your best friend. If you would, forgive yourself! Also, ask yourself whether you are trying to be perfect, demanding of yourself that you never make a mistake. Remember, if you don't make mistakes, you will not learn. Think of babies learning to walk, and consider how often they fall before they can walk confidently. Mistakes are educational, if you analyse them carefully, so that the same error is not repeated.

Your emotional health will improve with an increase of self-esteem. How does one increase this precious commodity? Become aware of how you are affected by those who put you down, and avoid them when possible. Seek out those who value you – they are friends indeed. Our conditioning can make us devalue ourselves, by making us live our lives according to others rules. These rules may not have been intended to have a negative effect, but may have become redundant in a quickly changing society. If a person becomes consciously aware of their conditioning. Then they are free to review it, and decide whether it is valuable or restricting.

Also, be aware of negative thoughts you may have towards yourself (the monkey on your shoulder), so you can learn to challenge them. To demonstrate the effectiveness of a positive attitude, try it for a month. Say nothing negative. Try praise at every appropriate opportunity, but never falsely. People are afraid of "spoiling" others and neglect to prize them.

Remember to treat yourself occasionally and make time to do the things that you enjoy.

References

Introduction

(1) *British Medical Journal*, 23 April 1955 (Supplement), pp. 190–3.

(2) Waxman, D., 1989, *Hartland's Medical and Dental Hypnosis*, Balliere-Tindall.

(3) Wilber, K. and G., 1991, *Grace and Grit*, New York, Gill and MacMillan page 43. (Quoting New York Times 24 April 1988).

(4) Seliger, S., 1984, *Stop Killing Yourself*, Exly Pub. Ltd, p. 18.

Chapter One

(1) Van Pelt, S.J., 1950, *Hypnosis and the Power Within*, London: Skeffington, Chapter 1.

(2) Waxman, D., 1989, *Hartland's Medical and Dental Hypnosis* (3rd ed.) Bailliere-Tindall.

(3) Mesmer F. A., 1971, *Le Magnetisme Animal* (ed. R. Amadou), Paris: Payot, p. 139.

(4) Braid, J., 1899, *Neurypnology or the Rationale of Nervous Sleep Considered in Relation with Animal Magnetism*, London, Redway.

(5) Waxman, D., *op. cit.*, p. 9.

(6) Esdaile, J., 1856, *The Introduction of Mesmerism ... into the Public Hospitals of India*, London: W. Kent, 2nd ed., p. 40.

(7) Waxman, D., *op. cit.*, pp. 10–11.

(8) Bernheim, H., 1899, *Suggestive Therapeutics*, (trans. CA Herter), GP Putnam's Sons, New York.

(9) Charcot, J.M., 1890, *Oeuveres Completes,* Metallotherapic et Hypnotism, Bournevill *et al.,* Brissaud, Paris.

(10) Charcot J.M., 1877, *Lectures on the Diseases of the Nervous System,* London, New Sydenham Society.

(11) Freud, S., Breuer, J., 1991, *Studies on Hysteria,* Penguin Books, p. 88.

(12) *Ibid.,* pp. 36, 172.

(13) Jung, C.G., 1964, *Memories, Dreams, Reflections,* Readers' Union, Collins and Routledge and Kegan Paul, London, pp. 131–2.

(14) Forel, A., 1906, *Hypnotism or Suggestion and Psychotherapy,* London: Rebman, pp. 219–20.

(15) Erickson, M.H., 1941, *Hypnosis: A General Review,* Diseases of the Nervous System, 2, pp. 13–18.

(16) Haley J., 1986, *Uncommon Therapy.* London, WW Norton & Co. Ltd.

(17) Grinder, J. & Bandler, R., 1981, *Trance-formations, Neuro-Linguistic Programming & the Structure of Hypnosis,* Real People Press, p. 3.

(18) Chong D. K., 1987, Personal Communication to D. Waxman, *Hartland's Medical and Dental Hypnosis* (3rd ed.) Bailliere Tindall, 1989, p. 262.

(19) Kroger, W.S., 1977, *Clinical and Experimental Hypnosis,* (2nd ed.). Philadelphia: JB Lippincott Company, p. 10.

(20) Levant, R.F., Shlien, J.M., 1984, *Client Centered Therapy and the Person Centred Approach.* Prager. New York, p. 313.

(21) Spanos, N.P., Barber, T.X., 1974, "Toward a Convergence in Hypnosis Research", *American Psychologists,* 29, pp. 500–11.

(22) Hilgard, E.R. and Hilgard, J.R., 1975, *Hypnosis in the Relief of Pain,* Los Altos, CA: Karfman.

(23) Hilgard, E.R., 1965, *Hypnotic Susceptibility,* New York: Harcourt, Brace & World.

(24) Orne, M.T., 1977, "The Construct of Hypnosis: Implications of the Definition for Research and Practice". *Annals of the New York Academy of Sciences,* 296, 1–314.

(25) Blake, H., Genrard, R.W., 1937, "Brain Potentials During Sleep". *American Journal of Physiology*, 119, pp. 692–703.

(26) Barber, T.X., 1969, *Hypnosis: A Scientific Approach*, New York, Von Nostrand, Reinhold.

(27) BBC2 film "Hypnosis, Can Your Mind Control Your Body?" By Michael Barnes, 27 September 1982.

(28) Barber, J., 1977, Rapid Induction Analgesia: A Clinical Report. *American Journal of Clinical Hypnosis*, 19, pp 138–147.

(29) Gindes, B.C., 1953, *New Concepts of Hypnosis*. George Allen & Unwin, London, p. 77.

(30) Galin, D. Implications for Psychiatry of Left and Right Cerebral Specialization: A Neurophysiological Context for Unconscious Processes. *Archives of General Psychiatry*, 31, pp. 572–83.

(31) Wickramasekera, 1988, *Clinical and Behavioral Medicine*, Plenum Press, New York & London. p. 119.

(32) Rogers, C.R., 1951, *Client-Centered Therapy*, Constable and Co. Books Ltd., pp. 64–78.

(33) Weitzenhoffer, A.M., 1957, *General Techniques of Hypnotism, Grune and Stratton*, Inc., New York, p. 61.

(34) *Ibid.*, Ref 2, p. 47.

(35) Kroger, W.S., 1977, *Clinical and Experimental Hypnosis* (2nd ed.), J. B. Lippincott Company, p. 10.

(36) Rogers, C.R. Paper for: The Foundations of the Person-Centred Approach. Centre for Studies of the Person, La Jolla, California 90237, pp. 104–105.

(37) Ferguson, M., 1979, Special Issue: Prigogine's, Science of Becoming, *Brain/Mind Bulletin*, 4, No. 13, 21 May. In C.R. Rogers, Paper for: The Foundations of the Person-Centred Approach. Centre for Studies of the Person, La Jolla, California 90237, pp. 105–106.

(38) Watson, J.B., 1913, Psychology as the Behaviourist Views it, *Psychology Review*, 20, pp. 158–177.

(39) Waxman, *op. cit.*, p. 15.

(40) Wolpe, J., 1958, *Psychotherapy by Reciprocal Inhibition*, Stanford University Press, Stanford, California.

(41) Atkinson, R.L. *et al.*, 1990, *Introduction to Psychology* (10th Ed.; International ed.), Harcourt, Brace, Jovanovich. pp. 64–78.

(42) Zeig, J.K., 1987, *The Evolution of Psychotherapy*. New York: Brunner Mazel.

Chapter Two

(1) Martin, P., 1997, *The Sickening Mind*, HarperCollins.

(2) Green, E. & A., 1977, *Beyond Biofeedback*, New York, Delta.

(3) Miller, H.B., 1970, "Your emotions: can they influence disease?", *Science Digest*, July, pp. 61–64.

(4) Hypnosis and Healing (BBC television documentary, 1981).

(5) La Baw, W.L., 1970, "Regular Use of Suggestibility by Pediatric Bleeders", *Haematologia*, pp. 419–25.

(6) La Baw, W. *et al.*, 1975, "The use of self-hypnosis with children with cancer, *American Journal of Clinical Hypnosis*, 4, Vol. 17, April.

(7) Goldberg, J.G., 1981, *Psychotherapeutic Treatment of Cancer Patients*, Free Press, pp 64–70.

(8) Goldberg, B., 1985, "The Treatment of Cancer Through Hypnosis". *Psychology: A Quarterly Journal of Human Behaviour*, Vol. 22, Part no. 3–4, pp. 36–9.

(9) Cangello, V.W., 1961/2, *American Journal of Clinical Hypnosis*, vol. 4, pp. 215–26.

(10) Newton, B.W. "Use of Hypnosis in the Treatment of Cancer Patients", *American Journal of Clinical. Hypnosis*, Vol. 25, No. 2–3, Oct., pp. 82–3.

(11) Eliseo, T.S., 1974, "Three Examples of Hypnosis in the Treatment of Organic Brain Syndrome with Psychosis". *International Journal of Clinical and Experimental Hypnosis*, Vol. 22, 1, pp. 9–19.

(12) Margolis, C.G., 1982, Hypnotic Imagery with Cancer Patients", *American. J. Clinical. Hypnosis*, Vol. 25, pp. 2–3, Oct.–Jan. 83, pp. 128–134.

(13) Miller, H.B., 1970, "Your Emotions: Can They Influence Disease?", *Science Digest*, July, pp. 61–4.

(14) Meares, A., 1976, "Regression of Cancer After Intensive Meditation", *Medical Journal of Australia*, Vol. 2, p. 184.

(15) Meares, A., 1979, "Regression of Cancer of the Rectum Following Intensive Meditation", *Medical Journal of Australia*, pp. 539–40.

(16) Meares, A., 1980, "Remission of Undifferentiated Carcinoma of the Lung Associated with Intensive Meditation", *Journal of the American Society of Psychosomatic Dentistry and Medicine*, Vol. 27, No. 2.

(17) Meares, A., 1981, Regression of Recurrence of the Carcinoma of the Breast of Mastectomy Site Associated with Intensive Meditation, *Australian Family Physician*, Vol. 10, pp. 218–219.

(18) Meares, A., 1978, Regression of Osteogenic Sarcoma Metastases Associated with Intensive Meditation, *The Medical Journal of Australia*, 2, p. 433. 21 Oct.

(19) Meares, A., 1961, What Makes the Patient Better, *Lancet*, 10 June, pp. 1280–1.

(20) Campbell, P. and Jean-Roche, L., 1983, Hypnosis, Surgery and Mind-Body Interaction an Historical Evaluation, *Canadian J of Behavioural Sci.* vol. 15, Part 4, Oct. 1, pp. 351–72.

(21) Elliotson, J., 1977, *Numerous Cases of Surgical Operation Without Pain*, Robinson G. N. (ed.), Significant Contributions to the History of Psychology, 1750–1920. Series A, Vol. X, Washington, D.C., University Publications of America. (Originally published 1843.)

(22) Elliotson, J., 1848, Cure of a true cancer of the female breast with Mesmerism, *Zoist* 23, Vol. 23, p. 312.

(23) Janet, P., 1925, *Psychological Healing*, vols 1 & 2, London, George Allen & Unwin.

Chapter Three

(1) Schoen, M., 1993, "Resistance to Health", *American Journal of Clinical Hypnosis*, 36, Vol. 1, pp. 47–54.

(2) Levenson, F.B., 1985, *The Causes and Prevention of Cancer*, Sidgewick and Jackson.

(3) Bahnson, C.B., 1980, "Stress and Cancer", Part 1, *Psychosomatics*, December, 12, Vol. 21, pp. 975–81.

(4) Goleman, D., 1995, *Emotional Intelligence*, Bloomsbury, Refs 27, 46, Chapter 11, pp. 174 & 180–1.

(5) Schneck, Penn, De-Novo, 1971, "Brain Tumours in Renal Transplant Recipients", *Lancet*, 1, pp. 983–6.

(6) Kersey and Spector, 1975, *Immune and Deficiency Diseases In Persons at High Risk of Cancer*, New York, Academic Press.

(7) Araoz, D.L., 1983/4, "Use of Hypnotic Techniques with Oncology Patients", *Journal of Psychosocial Oncology*, 4, Vol. 1, Winter.

(8) La Baw, W. *et al.*, 1975, "The Use of Self-Hypnosis with Children with Cancer", *American Journal of Clinical Hypnosis*, Vol. 17, 4 April.

(9) Ruch, J.C., 1975, "Self-hypnosis : The Result of Heterohypnosis or Vice Versa", *International Journal of Clinical & Experimental Hypnosis*, 4, Vol. 23, pp. 282–304.

(10) Jackobs, T.J., Charles, E., 1980, "Life Events and the Occurrence of Cancer in Children", *Psychosomatic Medicine*, 1, Vol. 42, January.

(11) Zeitzer, L.K. and LeBaron, S. (1983) *Behavioural Medicine Update*, Vol. 5, Parts 2–3, Autumn, pp. 17–22.

(12) Meares, A., 1961, "What Makes the Patient Better", *Lancet*, 10 June, p. 1280–1.

(13) Meares, A. Form of Intensive Meditation Associated with the Regression of Cancer, *American Journal of Clinical Hypnosis*. Vol. 25, No. 2–3, Oct. 82–Jan. 83

(14) *The Zoist*, Vol. 23. October 1848, p. 213.

(15) *Hartland's Medical and Dental Hypnosis* (3rd ed.), Bailliere Tindall, 1989.

(16) Ananand, B., China, G., Singh, B., 1961, *EEG Journal*.

(17) Banquet, J.P., 1973, "Spectral Analyses of the EEG in Education", *Electroencephalographic Clinical Neurophysiology*, August: No. 35(2): pp. 143–151.

(18) Rossi, E.L., Cheek, D.B., *Mind Body Therapy*, WW Norton & Co. N.Y., London, ISBN, 0-393-70052-6.

(19) Zeig, J.K. 1987, *The Evolution of Psychotherapy*. New York: Brunner Mazel.

(20) Hall, H.R. "Hypnosis and the Immune System, A Review with Implications for cancer and the Psychology of Healing". *American Journal of Clinical Hypnosis*, Vol. 25, Nos 2–3, Oct. '82–Jan. '83.

(21) Mason, A.A., 1952, *British Medical Journal*, Vol. 2, pp. 422–3.

(22) BBC, *Horizon*, 1997.

(23) Goldberg, B., 1985, The Treatment of Cancer through Hypnosis, *Psychology a Quarterly Journal of Human Behaviour*, Vol. 22, 3/4, pp. 36–39.

(24) Levenson, J.A. & Bemis, C., 1991, "The Role of Psychological Factors in Cancer Onset & and Progression". *Psychosomatics*, Vol. 32, No. 2, Spring.

Chapter Four

(1) Finkelstein, S., Howard, M.G., "Cancer Prevention – A Three Year Study", *A. J. Clin. Hypnosis*, Vol. 25, No 2–3, Oct. '82–Jan. '83, p. 177

(2) Shapiro, A.K, Morris, L.A., 1978, *"The Placebo Effect in Medical and Psychological Therapies"*, in *The Handbook of Psychotherapy and Behaviour Change*, Ganfield SL, Bergin AE (eds), John Wiley & Sons, New York, pp. 369–410.

(3) Grunbaum, A., 1981, The Placebo Concept. *Behav. Res. Ther.* 19: 157–67.

(4) Grunbaum, A., 1986, The Placebo Concept in Medicine and Psychiatry, *Psychol. Med.*, 16: 19–38.

(5) Lowinger, P. & Dobie, S., 1968, "What Makes the Placebo Work?", *Archives of General Psychiatry* 20, pp. 84–88.

(6) Lowinger, P. 1963, "Evaluation of Mephenoxalone in a Single and Double-Blind Design", *Amer. J. Psychiat.*, 120, 66–67, July.

(7) Beecher H., 1955, "The Powerful Placebo", JAMA 159; 1602–1606 (Dec 24) in: Rickel K. (Ed) "Nonspecific Factors of Drug Therapy". Springfield, 111: Charles C. Thomas, 1968.

(8) Brown, W.A., 1998, The Placebo Effect, *Scientific American*, January, pp. 68–73.

(9) Martin, P., 1997, *The Sickening Mind*, HarperCollins.

(10) *Watchdog*, BBC1, 17 June 1996.

(11) Goldberg, J.G., 1981, *Psychotherapeutic Treatment of Cancer Patients*, The Free Press.

(12) Peek, C.J., 1977, "A Critical Look at the Theory of Placebo", *Biofeedback & Self-Regulation*, 2, pp. 327–35.

(13) Frank, J.D., 1961, *Persuasion and Healing*, Baltimore, Johns Hopkins Press.

(14) Kirsch, I., 1985, Response Expectancy as a Determinant of Experience and Behaviour. *American Psychologist*, 40, 1189–1202.

(15) Evans, F.J. & McGlashan, T.H. Specific & Nonspecific Factors in Hypnotic Analgesia: A reply to Wagstaff, *British Journal of Clinical & Experimental Hypnosis* 4, 141–147.

(16) Orne, M.T., 1974, *Pain Suppression by Hypnosis & Related Phenomena*. In J.J. Bonical (ed.) *Pain*, New York: Raven press.

(17) Evans, F.J., 1990, Hypnosis & Pain Control *Australian Journal of Clinical & Experimental Hypnosis*, Vol. 18, No. 1, pp. 21–33.

(18) Spanos, N.P. *et al.*, 1989, Hypnosis, Suggestion & Placebo in the Reduction of Experimental Pain, *Journal of Abnormal Psychology*, Vol. 98, No. 3, 285–293.

(19) Higard, E.R. & Hilgard, J.R., 1983, *Hypnosis in the Relief of Pain*, (2nd ed.), Los Altos, CA; William Kaufmann.

(20) Sturpp, H.J. *et al.*, 1974, Effects of Suggestion on Total Respiratory Resistance in Mild Asthmatics. *Journal of Psychosomatic Research*, 18, pp. 337–346.

(21) White, L. *et al.*, 1985, *Placebo Theory, Research and Mechanism*. New York: Guildford. (Note by F.J. Evans.)

(22) Eysenck, H.J., 1989, "Personality, Primary & Secondary Suggestibility, & Hypnosis", in Gheorghiu, V.A. *et al.* (eds), *Suggestibility: Theory & Research* (57–68), Berlin: Stringer-Verlag.

(23) McGlasham, T.H. *et al.*, 1969, "The Nature of Hypnotic Analgesia & Placebo Response to Experimental Pain", *Psychosomatic Medicine*, 31, pp. 227–46.

(24) Orne, M.T., 1974, "Pain Suppression by Hypnosis & Related Phenomena", in J.J. Bonica (ed.), *Pain*, New York: Raven.

(25) Evans, F.J. *et al.*, "Sleep Induced Behavioral Response: Relationships to Susceptibility to Hypnosis & Laboratory Sleep Patterns", *Journal of Nervous & Mental Disease*, pp. 148, 169 and 467–76.

(26) Bernheim, H., *Hypnosis & Suggestion in Psychotherapy*, New York: University Books (originally published in 1888).

(27) Bowers, K.S, 1976, *Hypnosis for the Seriously Curious*, Monterey, CA: Brooks/Coles

(28) Hilgard, E.R., 1973, "The Domain of Hypnosis: With Comments on Alternative Paradigms", *American Psychologists*, 23, pp. 972–82.

(29) Barber, T.X. & Calvery, D.S., 1964, "The Definition of the Situation as a Variable Affecting 'Hypnotic Like' Suggestibility", *Journal of Clinical Psychology*, 20, 438–40.

(30) Rosental, D. & Framl, J.D., 1956, "Psychotherapy and the Placebo Effect", *Psychol. Bull*, 53, 294–302.

(31) Plansky, N. & Kovnin, J., 1956, "Clients Reactions to Initial Interviews", *Human Relations*, 9, 237–242.

(32) Brill, N.Q. & Storrow, H.W, 1963, "Pronastic Factors in Psychotherapy", *Journal of the American Medical Association*, 183.

(33) Hiller, F.W., 1958, "An Analysis of Patient–Therapist Compatibility", *Journal of Consulting Psychology*, 22, 341–353.

(34) Lowinger, P. & Dobie, S., 1964, "Psychiatrists Variable in the Process of Interview & Treatment", *Nature*, 201, 1246–1247.

(35) Goldstein, A.P., 1962, *Therapist–Patient Expectancies in Psychotherapy*, New York: Pergamon Press.

(36) Cartwright, D.S., 1958, "Faith & Improvement in Psychotherapy", *Journal of Counselling Psychology*, 5, 174–177.

(37) Lieberman, L.R. & Dunlop, J.T., 1979, O'Leary & Barovec's "Conceptualization of Placebo: The Placebo Paradox", *American Psychologist*, 34, pp. 553–4.

(38) Gindes, B.C., 1951, *New Concepts of Hypnosis*, George Allen & Unwin, London. pp. 77, 78. *Hartland's Medical and Dental Hypnosis* (3rd ed.), Balliere-Tindall, 1989.

(39) Hartland, J. & Waxman, D., 1989, *Hartland's Medical and Dental Hypnosis*, Bailliene Tindall (3rd ed.), p. 9.

(40) Mesmer, F.A., 1971, *Le Magnetismic Animal* (ed. R. Amadou), Paris: Payot, p. 139.

(41) Ruch, J.C., 1975, "Self-hypnosis: The Result of Heterohypnosis or Vice Versa", *The International Journal of Clinical & Experimental Hypnosis*, Vol. 23, 4, pp. 282–304.

(42) Shea, J.D., 1991, *Suggestion, Placebo & Expectation: Immune Effects & Other Bodily Change*, Human Suggestibility, J. F. Schumaker, Routledge, pp. 270–1.

Chapter Five

(1) Personal Communication.

(2) Maltz M., 1960, *Psycho-Cybernetics*, Prentice-Hall, pp. 47–49.

Chapter Six

(1) Forel, A., 1906, *Hypnotism or Suggestion and Psychotherapy*, London: Rebman, pp. 219–20.

(2) Personal Communication.

(3) BBC2, *Hypnosis and Healing*.

(4) Leboyer, F., 1991, *Birth Without Violence*, Mandarin.

(5) Vernay, T. & Kelly, J., 1981, *The Secret Life of the Unborn Child*, Warner Books.

Chapter Seven

(1) Axline V., 1964, *Dibs In Search of Self*, Penguin Books.

(2) Miller, A., 1991, Training Childhood. *Trauma in Creativity and Destructiveness*. Anchor Books.

(3) Rogers, Carl, 1961, *On Becoming a Person: A Psychotherapist's View of Psychotherapy*, London: Constable.

(4) Jackson, D., 1989, *Three in a Bed*, Bloomsbury.

(5) Stanton and Oakley, "Patterns of Illnesses before Cot Deaths". *Archives of Diseases in Childhood*, Vol. 58, pp. 878–81.

(6) Leidloft, J., 1975, *Continuum Concept*, Futura.

(7) Miller, Alice, 1991, *Breaking Down the Wall of Silence – to join the waiting child*, Virago.

Index